DOCTOR HOMOLA'S FAT-DISINTEGRATOR DIET

DOCTOR HOMOLA'S FAT-DISINTEGRATOR DIET

Samuel Homola, D. C.

Foreword by Joseph L. Kaplowe, M. D.

Art Work by Bibiana Neal

Parker Publishing Company, Inc.

West Nyack, New York

Library of Congress Cataloging in Publication Data

Homola, Samuel.
    Doctor Homola's fat-disintegrator diet.

    Includes index.
    1. Reducing diets. 2. Food, Natural. 3. Reducing
exercises. I. Title.
RM222.2.H585   613.2'5   76-22189
ISBN 0-13-216325-X

Printed in the United States of America

DEDICATED TO

Jimmy and Betty Rowell
Lee and Marcella Brown
Edrie and Beverly Hunt
Ronald and Shirley Thayer

The type of friends who come along once in a lifetime.

Books by Samuel Homola

Bonesetting, Chiropractic, and Cultism
Backache: Home Treatment and Prevention
Muscle Training for Athletes
A Chiropractor's Treasury of Health Secrets
La Salud Y Sus Secretos
Secrets of Naturally Youthful Health and Vitality
Doctor Homola's Natural Health Remedies
Doctor Homola's Life-Extender Health Guide
Doctor Homola's Fat-Disintegrator Diet

FOREWORD
BY A DOCTOR OF MEDICINE

Many books have been written on how to reduce body fat. Most of them deal with fad aspects of dieting that present unbalanced diets that are often dangerous or detrimental to health. Doctor Homola has written one of the few books that can truly be called a uniquely safe and effective approach to reducing bodyweight.

Faithfully adhering to the use of the seven basic natural food groups as recommended by Doctor Homola in this book will improve your health as well as get rid of excess body fat. Doctor Homola's diet plan is, in fact, so sensible and so effective that every overweight man or woman can safely follow the same basic diet plan with uniformly good results.

In my many years of medical practice, I have seen examples of the dangers of overweight. I have also witnessed the harmful effects of unscientific reducing diets. There is no doubt in my mind that this latest book by Doctor Homola is an outstanding contribution offering a real solution to the problem of overweight. I recommend it to you without reservation. Reading it will change your life, and the guidance it offers will solve your weight problem once and for all.

Joseph L. Kaplowe, M.D.

WHAT THIS BOOK CAN DO
FOR YOU

When Marcus C. first stepped onto the scales in my office, he weighed 210 pounds at a height of five feet and eight inches. Shortness of breath, fatigue, and other symptoms of aging constantly reminded him of the progressive deterioration that was taking place in his body. His blood cholesterol was much too high for a forty-year-old man, and he was a borderline diabetic.

"I've been fat since my senior year in college," Marcus confessed, "and I just keep getting fatter. None of the diets I've tried seem to work. The last time I went on a diet, I developed gout, and my doctor told me to quit eating meat. I'm really confused about this diet business."

Like most people who have trouble controlling their bodyweight, Marcus did not eat properly when he was not on a diet. When he did go on a diet, he usually chose one of the fad diets that could not be followed for more than a few weeks at a time without harmful effects. I explained the essentials of good nutrition to Marcus and then outlined a couple of basic rules for him to follow. I did *not* give him a diet that listed the foods he should eat at every meal.

With a few simple instructions, Marcus began losing his excess body fat with no trouble at all. And he continued to do so without any further special instructions. There was no starvation and no weakness. After six months of eating *normally,* Marcus had no obvious body fat, and his health had improved considerably.

Chances are you can solve your overweight problem with the same simple procedures that Marcus followed. You can get started *now* by reading Chapter 1 of this book.

REDUCING CAN SAVE YOUR LIFE

Overweight is a common problem in the United States. More than one-half of the population over the age of forty is too fat. Excessive use of refined and processed foods contributes to a build-up of body fat that plays a major role in the development of many serious and fatal diseases. Diabetes, arthritis, heart disease, hardened arteries, high blood pressure, cancer, kidney ailments, varicose veins, hernia, gallbladder trouble, and other common ailments are often related to obesity. Surgery can be complicated by layers of fat that require deeper and longer incisions. Strains placed on muscles and joints as a result of overweight cause aches and pains that range from aching feet to a throbbing headache. No part of the body escapes the burden of fat.

Being "fat" has many personal and cosmetic disadvantages. Clothing does not fit properly. Sexual activities are more difficult. The unattractive appearance of a fat, flabby body may actually repel attention from the opposite sex. Business and social activities may also suffer. Many people tend to think that an obese person is a glutton with no courage or willpower. As a result, fat people are often ignored in social and professional circles.

WITH MY DIET, REDUCING FAT IS SAFE AND SIMPLE

Most fat people are overweight because they do not eat the proper foods rather than because they overeat. This means that *proper selection and preparation of foods* can eliminate the problem of overweight, thus preventing disease, relieving aches and pains, and restoring the youthful health you need to feel good and look good.

All this can be accomplished simply by *eliminating processed foods and substituting a variety of fresh, natural foods.* Using my method of combining the basic natural foods, you can literally *disintegrate* excess body fat without starving or counting calories. You can lose three or four pounds a week with no trouble at all, without even going on a diet. Excess body fat will disappear as if by magic—as if some invisible ray were disintegrating the fat while you eat to your heart's content. Sound too good to be true? The secret lies in combining a balanced variety of *natural* foods, so that your body can normalize its weight the way nature intended.

YOU CAN IMPROVE YOUR HEALTH
WHILE REDUCING YOUR WEIGHT

With my fat-disintegrator diet, you can improve your health while shedding pounds of excess body fat. You can be slimmer, happier, and healthier without the risk or the sacrifice associated with the type of diet that requires a doctor's supervision. Once you get started on my diet, you'll want to stay on it for the rest of your life—and you can do so without outside help or supervision.

Actually, my fat-disintegrator diet is not a diet at all in the usual sense. It's simply a *guide* that allows you to use your own judgment in selecting the foods you eat. I simply tell you what *types* of foods to eat and how to prepare them. I want to make you so knowledgeable about eating that you won't need to follow a menu that tells you exactly what to eat at every meal. You'll *know* what to eat, and you won't be taken in by fad diets that damage your health.

My years of experience in training athletes and treating patients have revealed to me what I feel is the easiest and most effective method available to reduce body fat without depriving yourself or damaging your health. There is nothing mysterious about my diet. Everything I advise you to do is based on the latest scientific research. In my position as a special consultant to Peter Lupus Leisure Health World in Panama City, Florida, I must keep abreast of all the latest developments dealing with the subject of reducing bodyweight. So you can rest assured that my knowledge in this field is timely and up-to-date.

It's all here for your personal use. You can follow my eating guide without making a single visit to a doctor's office. All you have to do is keep this book handy so that you can refer to it frequently to refresh your memory about selecting and preparing foods.

Samuel Homola, D. C.

Table of Contents

How to Go On My Fat-Disintegrator Diet One Week at a Time (Cont.)

Have a Whole-Grain Product at Least Once Daily (44) . . . Use Skimmed Milk Products (45) . . . Fill Up with Green Salads (45) . . . Three Sample Menus for Daily Use (46) . . . Let Your Appetite Be Your Guide (48) . . . How to Alternate the Basic Food Groups (49) . . . Cook Once Each Day (50) . . . How to Cut Down on Calories without Counting Calories (51) . . . A Standard Low-Calorie Diet (53) . . . How to Prevent Side Effects by Controlling Carbohydrate (54) . . . A Diet Is Only a Guide (54) . . . Go Easy on Alcohol (55) . . . Will a Natural Foods Diet Work for You? (55) . . . Summary (56)

1

How You Can Disintegrate Excess Body Fat with Three Square Meals a Day

Everyone has to eat. Eating builds health and maintains life. It's also one of life's pleasures. Foods please the palate, satisfy craving, and ease the pains of hunger. No one wants to go on a starvation diet—and no one should. It's not necessary to go hungry in order to lose weight. Any diet that keeps you hungry is not an adequate diet, and it's likely to be deficient in essential nutrients. You cannot stay on such a diet for more than a few weeks without damaging your health.

If you eat properly, you can eat *plenty* and still reduce your bodyweight. It's simply a matter of selecting the right foods and then preparing them properly. If you eat a balanced diet of properly prepared *natural* foods, you may even eat *five times* a day instead of the customary three times if you like. Your body's built-in appetite mechanism will automatically let you know when you have eaten enough to satisfy your body's needs. Snacking between meals will very likely reduce your appetite so that you won't overeat at mealtime. You'll learn in another chapter of this book how such snacks will help keep your blood sugar at just the right level for maximum energy throughout the day.

The case of Claude D. is a good example of what happens when blood sugar fluctuates from one extreme to another. Claude had decided that the best way to reduce was to eat only two meals a day. He would have a light breakfast at home and then have an evening meal at the local cafeteria. He satisfied his craving during the day by drinking numerous cups of black coffee. "The coffee gives me the lift I need to keep going," he explained. When Claude sat down for his evening meal, he gorged himself with all kinds of refined and processed foods. The result was that he *gained* weight instead of losing. An abnormal elevation of blood sugar during the night forced his body to store the sugar as fat. And the coffee he had during the day further stimulated the storage of blood sugar as fat. I was not surprised when Claude told me that he had gained ten pounds in three weeks on such a diet.

When Claude switched to three light meals daily with between-meal snacks of fresh fruit, cottage cheese, and baked chicken, he lost weight slowly but steadily. He was actually eating *less* than when he had only one meal a day, and he was never hungry. The level of his blood sugar was consistent for the first time in years.

It may be that you, too, can reduce your bodyweight by eating more often than you normally do. Once you learn how to select and prepare your foods, you'll be able to reduce your bodyweight by eating *more* rather than less. Other chapters in this book will tell you everything you need to know about the foods you eat. In this chapter, you'll learn how you can shed pounds of fat simply by following certain basic rules and by eliminating certain types of foods. Be sure to study *all* of the chapters of this book, however, so that you can acquire the knowledge you need to eat for the best of health.

A GENERAL DIET IS BEST FOR MOST PEOPLE

Most "special" diets are either difficult to follow or nutritionally unbalanced. I do not believe that it's necessary to make out a list of specific foods to be eaten in measured amounts at each meal. It's enough to know what *types* of foods you should eat, so that you may simply select from available foods. If your diet allows you to eat lean meat, for example, you may eat any kind of meat that has had all the visible fat cut away. (Fish and poultry are best, as you'll learn later in this book.)

You can eat any kind of vegetable you want as long as you select one or two from each basic group each day—depending upon what vegetables are in season. Vegetables are usually classified in three groups: (1) green and yellow vegetables, (2) tomatoes and raw cabbage, and (3) potatoes and other vegetables.

You'll learn more about *all* the basic food groups in another chapter of this book. In the meantime, remember that it's very important to eat a variety of *natural* foods in order to prevent a nutritional deficiency that may cause an abnormal craving for high-calorie foods. If you eat properly, you can be healthy as well as lean.

THE DANGERS OF A BAD REDUCING DIET

Many popular reducing diets are unbalanced and dangerous. A diet that is too low in calories supplied by natural carbohydrate, for example, may upset body metabolism and result in a loss of protein from vital organs. High-fat diets may clog arteries with hard fat and cholesterol. There is now some evidence to indicate that too much fat in the diet may even cause cancer or contribute to premature aging.*

An all-meat diet may trigger a case of gout, overload the kidneys, and contribute to the formation of kidney stones. A low-protein diet can weaken muscles and organs. In addition to being deficient in protein and other essential nutrients, a vegetable diet can contribute to the development of anemia. Reducing diets that restrict natural carbohydrates and emphasize protein and fat deprive the intestinal tract of the

---

*"Nutrition and Health of Older People," Schlenker, et al., *The American Journal of Clinical Nutrition,* October, 1973.

cellulose and other fibers the bowels need to function normally. Lack of adequate vegetable and fruit fiber in the diet can lead to the development of constipation, diverticulitis, colon cancer, appendicitis, intestinal polyps, and other distressing bowel problems.

High-fat reducing diets are presently very popular. The side effects of these diets often force persons who use them to take laxatives to correct constipation, medicine to prevent attacks of gout, and salt with potassium to relieve muscle weakness caused by excessive loss of body fluids.

Any diet that eliminates one of the basic food groups or limits food selection to one type of food is likely to be deficient in essential vitamins and minerals. You can lose weight rapidly on such a diet, but you cannot stay on it for very long. And just as soon as the diet is discontinued, the lost fat creeps back.

You can lose weight safely and effectively on a properly balanced diet of *natural* foods. You can stay on such a diet for the rest of your life—without the rigid discipline of counting calories. It's simply a matter of eating properly.

NATURAL FOODS ARE NOT AS FATTENING AS REFINED FOODS

Marie B. weighed 180 pounds when she first began following my dietary recommendations. "I've been starving myself on a low-calorie diet for several weeks," she complained, "but I haven't lost more than a pound or two." I asked Marie to write down everything she ate for a week. When I looked at the list, I found that she ate small amounts of a great variety of processed foods. There were hidden calories in catsup, canned goods, TV dinners, and other foods that contained sugar, oil, or flour. When she eliminated *all* of the refined and processed foods in her diet and stuck to fresh, natural foods, she began to lose weight quite rapidly. *She lost 15 pounds the first month.* In less than six months, her weight was down to a slim, trim 115 pounds.

"I eat more than I have ever eaten," she exclaimed. "And I'm having no trouble keeping my weight down. This natural foods diet is great!"

There is now considerable evidence to indicate that the calories in a fresh, natural food are not as fattening as the calories in a refined or processed food. One reason for this is that refined foods contain a *simple* carbohydrate that is absorbed into the bloodstream so rapidly that it floods the blood with glucose. This overstimulates the pancreas, which releases a flood of insulin that stores an excessive amount of blood sugar as glycogen (much of which is converted to fat). A drop in blood sugar then results in a craving for sweets, much like the alcoholic's craving for alcohol. Artificial sweets and refined carbohydrates supply empty calories. And the combustion of empty calories in the body, like the combustion of alcohol, robs Peter to pay Paul, resulting in a deficiency of B vitamins and other nutrients.

The *complex* carbohydrates in natural foods are absorbed and assimilated more slowly, yielding nutrients and energy that can be utilized effectively by the body. You can snack on natural foods throughout the day without overeating, since your appetite mechanism and your blood sugar level, satisfied by a dependable source of nutrients, will prevent an abnormal craving for food. Natural foods also stay in the stomach longer, preventing the hunger pangs caused by an empty stomach.

If you eat the right foods, you can eat *more* and still lose weight. But you must limit your diet strictly to *natural* foods. *Persons who count calories on a diet that includes refined or processed foods may find it difficult or impossible to lose weight, even on a low-calorie diet.*

TEN SIMPLE RULES FOR REDUCING BODYWEIGHT

You'll learn more about how to lose weight safely and effectively in the remaining chapters of this book. In the meantime, you can begin losing weight *now* if you'll follow these simple rules:

(1) *Eliminate all foods containing sugar, white flour, or corn starch.* Remember that refined carbohydrates, such as candy, soft drinks, cake, spaghetti, pastries, and white bread, often trigger a pancreatic reaction that creates a craving for sweets and escalates the storage of body fat. With the average American consuming about 115 pounds of sugar a year along with great quantities of white flour, it's no wonder that overweight and obesity are so common. Many people could lose weight simply by cutting out sugar and its products.

(2) *Do not eat packaged snacks of any kind.* Every grocery store contains shelf after shelf of processed "snack foods" that are loaded with empty calories, harmful fat, and questionable additives. Don't buy them. Have a snack of cheese, fresh fruit, baked chicken, or some other natural food before you begin grocery shopping so that you won't be tempted to pick up a "convenient snack."

(3) *Concentrate upon eating lean meats, chicken, fish, eggs, fresh fruits and vegetables, raw salads, cottage cheese and yogurt made from skimmed milk, and whole-grain breads and cereals. Use skimmed milk, juices, and water as beverages.* If you are considerably overweight, leave off the bread and cereals for awhile. If fresh fruits do not satisfy your sweet tooth, eat a small amount of dried fruit *after* your regular meal. Remember, however, that dried fruits are fairly high in calories.

You'll learn in another chapter of this book how to prepare fat-fighting foods.

(4) *Make sure that the foods you eat are natural foods.* Always select *fresh* foods that have not been altered by a manufacturing or packing process. Everything you eat should be as close as possible to the form provided by nature. Foods processed for canning or packaging are usually deficient in nutrients and often contain sugar and other fattening or harmful additives.

(5) *Do not use butter, grease, or oil in preparing your foods.* Always roast, bake, or broil your meats. Cut out animal fat as much as possible. You'll get all the fat you need by using a small amount of vegetable oil on raw salads. (Linoleic acid is the most

essential of the fatty acids, since it cannot be manufactured by the body. Safflower oil is the best source of linoleic acid.)

(6) *Don't stuff yourself at mealtime.* Stop eating when you feel comfortably full. If you eat only natural foods, your appetite mechanism will let you know when you have had enough.

When you learn to eat smaller portions, so that you can get up from the table without feeling stuffed, you'll feel better and think better—and weight loss will be more rapid.

(7) *Snack between meals when you feel hungry.* If you get hungry between meals, eat a piece of baked chicken or a little cottage cheese with fresh fruit. A protein-rich snack between meals will keep your blood sugar up enough to prevent the craving that results in overeating at mealtime.

If you must constantly nibble on something to satisfy a nervous habit, keep a few raw vegetables handy, such as celery or carrot sticks. All kinds of fruits and vegetables supply bulk that helps curb the appetite by filling the stomach with indigestible fiber and cellulose.

(8) *Drink water when you are thirsty.* Don't get into the habit of drinking sweetened beverages when you are thirsty. Water will satisfy your thirst without contributing fattening calories or harmful additives. (I do not recommend the use of artificial sweeteners.)

(9) *Eat slowly* in order to give your body time to satisfy your hunger by absorbing nutrients. If you eat rapidly or bolt your food, your appetite mechanism won't have a chance to let you know when you have eaten enough to satisfy the needs of your body.

(10) *Be patient.* Don't get discouraged if weight loss seems slow. If you'll continue to eat properly, you'll eventually lose all of your excess body fat. Remember that you're eating for better health as well as to lose weight.

TAKE THE NEXT STEP

The basic rules outlined in this chapter are very general and can apply to anyone, overweight or not. The idea is to eat properly and see if your bodyweight will normalize itself. Persons who are obese and must lose weight more rapidly than someone who is only a little overweight will find more detailed information and stricter rules in other chapters of this book.

To repeat: No matter how much you weigh, you should study *all* of the material in this book so that you'll have the knowledge you need to control your weight and protect your health. So be sure to take the next step and begin reading Chapter 2.

SUMMARY

1. If you eat properly, you can improve your health as well as reduce your bodyweight.

2. Eliminating refined and processed foods from your diet is an important key to successful and permanent weight loss.

3. A balanced diet of *natural* foods, with a minimum amount of animal fat, will usually automatically adjust your bodyweight.

4. If your meals are made up of properly prepared natural foods, you can reduce your bodyweight and still eat snacks between meals.

5. The fat-disintegrator "diet" recommended in this book is an eating *guide* that you can follow for the rest of your life— without counting calories or going hungry.

2

The Role of
Fat-Disintegrator Foods
in Total Body Health

There are many reasons why foods that make people fat also make them unhealthy. Refined and processed foods that are rich in calories and deficient in nutrients, for example, are often totally lacking in the fiber or roughage your bowels need to function normally. Cancer of the colon, which is the second most common cause of death from malignancy, is now believed to be caused largely by inadequate fiber in the diet. Appendicitis, intestinal polyps, and diverticulitis are also common among persons who eat refined and processed foods. The reason for this, of course, is that such foods have had all their roughage removed in the refining process, so that nothing remains but soft, sticky bulk. This diet allows the bowels to become packed and clogged with waste that is difficult for the bowels to move. As a result, the waste stays in the lower bowel much longer than it should, allowing bacterial activity to produce cancer-causing toxins. Also, increased pressure in the lower bowel produces tiny ballooned-out pouches that often become inflamed and infected. The constipation that results inflames the appendix and produces polyps. Straining to empty a constipated bowel can greatly aggravate hemorrhoids. *All of this is caused by the same foods that commonly cause overweight.*

NATURAL FOODS ARE THE ANSWER!

If you eat fresh, *natural* foods, you'll get all the fiber your bowels need to function normally. You'll be able to *prevent* many of the diseases that commonly occur among "civilized people" who eat factory-prepared foods. Best of all, you'll be able to *eat more* without getting fat. The fiber or cellulose in natural foods supplies filling bulk with fewer calories—and the calories are not so easily absorbed. When you eat whole-grain bread, for example, only 86 percent of the calories in the bread are absorbed. But when you eat white bread, 97 percent of the calories are absorbed. The concentrated carbohydrate in white bread is, in fact, absorbed so rapidly that a sudden increase in blood sugar results in a pancreatic reaction that *lowers* blood sugar and creates a craving for sweets. This means that in addition to developing bowel diseases, persons on a diet that is high in refined carbohydrates often become *fat and fatigued.*

Refined cereals, packaged snacks, white-flour products, and similar foods have the same effect on blood sugar as white bread and refined sweets. If you're overweight, you should avoid them as if they were poison. You can truthfully say that you are "allergic" to refined carbohydrates, since they trigger a vicious cycle of hypoglycemia, fatigue, craving, and a build-up of body fat. One of my patients succinctly expressed his allergy to refined carbohydrates when he said, "Doc, I break out in *fat* when I eat bread and sweets."

FRESH FRUITS AND VEGETABLES
SUPPLY VALUABLE BULK

All types of fruits and vegetables contain fiber or cellulose that will keep the bowels healthy and help combat overweight. Whole-grain products, such as breads and cereals, contain bran, a form of roughage that also improves bowel health. Oatmeal, brown rice, cornmeal, and wheat are good sources of bran. Simply adding two or three tablespoons of pure bran to your diet each day will improve your general health by aiding your bowels. Try adding one tablespoonful to each meal.

The cellulose found in fresh fruits and vegetables actually sweeps the bowels clean, just like the action of a straw broom. Cellulose also holds moisture, so that stools will be soft and moist. So it's *very important* to eat some raw fruits and vegetables each day.

Between-meal snacks of raw fruits and vegetables will convey four important benefits: (1) reduce your appetite by filling your stomach with low-calorie bulk, (2) keep your blood sugar at a normal, consistent level, (3) supply moisture-retaining cellulose that will aid normal bowel function, and (4) supply essential vitamins and minerals along with the natural carbohydrate you need for energy.

Remember that you need a certain amount of indigestible matter in your diet. So don't worry about digesting everything you eat. You should always eat the pulp of fresh fruits and vegetables. Don't use juicing machines that separate the juice from the pulp. Juice without the pulp simply concentrates the calories and deprives you of filling bulk. If you have a digestive problem that won't permit you to swallow coarse fibers, use a blender that liquifies the entire fruit or vegetable—skin and all.

Even if you aren't interested in reducing your bodyweight or preventing obesity, your health and your body can benefit from eating the types of foods I recommend in my fat-disintegrator diet.

Many of my patients report an almost immediate improvement in bowel function after including raw fruits and vegetables in their diet. Christina A., for example, had suffered from chronic constipation for several years. Her bowels moved normally, however, after only one week of "dieting." It took only three months to shed 20 pounds and reduce her bodyweight to an attractive 120 pounds.

"My husband takes me out a lot more than he used to," Christina confided, "and things are a lot better at home. I had no idea that an improvement in my physical appearance would mean so much to my husband."

PROTECT YOUR ARTERIES WHILE YOU REDUCE FAT

Most medical men believe that the hard fat and cholesterol supplied by animal fats play a large part in the development of hardened arteries or atherosclerosis. There is also considerable evidence to indicate that sugar and refined carbohydrates contribute to a build-up of blood fat that clogs and hardens arteries. Triglycerides, for example, are a form of hard fat that is formed largely by refined carbohydrates. So in your efforts to protect your arteries and control your bodyweight, you'll have to avoid foods containing sugar and white flour as well as those animal products that are rich in hard fat and cholesterol.

How Cecil T. Reduced His Blood Cholesterol on a Reducing Diet

One of my patients, Cecil T., weighed 240 pounds on his 35th birthday. At a height of five feet, eleven inches, he was about 77 pounds overweight. Since he complained of fatigue and other vague symptoms, I had his blood tested and found that his cholesterol was elevated to 350 milligrams per 100 milliliters of blood—considerably above a safe level. His blood pressure and blood sugar were also too high. After several months on a natural foods reducing diet that eliminated sugar and white flour and cut animal fat to a minimum, Cecil lost 50 pounds. His blood pressure, blood sugar, and cholesterol dropped to a safe level, indicating a significant improvement in health.

"Getting rid of all that fat has changed my life," Cecil told me during an office visit. "I feel better than I have felt in years. And I owe it all to you."

"You did it all yourself," I responded. "If you'll continue to eat properly, you'll never have an overweight problem again. And you'll live a longer, healthier life."

If you follow the instructions outlined in this book, you, too, will experience the improvement in health that accompanies loss of excess body fat.

How to Cut Down on Fat-Forming, Artery-Hardening Animal Fat

One of the first things you should do to get rid of the harmful saturated fat in your diet is to cut away all the visible fat on the meat you eat—*before* you cook the meat. Whenever possible, bake or broil your meats over a slotted broiling pan so that fat cooked out of the meat can drip into a bottom pan for disposal.

If you boil meat in soup, always chill the soup so that you can skim off the hard surface fat. You may then rewarm the soup just before serving. You'll learn more about how to prepare foods when you read Chapter 4.

You need a certain amount of fat in your diet for good health. Lean meats contain a considerable amount of hidden fat. If you include meat in your diet, you'll get all the fat you need. Just to make sure that you don't get too much saturated fat, you should eat chicken or fish whenever you have a choice. They are just as rich in protein and nutrients as beef or pork, and they contain less saturated fat. You can eat chicken and fish every day if you like.

Cottage cheese and other skim milk products are good sources of low-fat protein. They contain only a small amount of saturated fat, so they can often be substituted for meat.

The *unsaturated* fat found in vegetable oil helps combat hardening and clogging of the arteries by diluting and softening hard or saturated fat. This is why some doctors recommend that you use vegetable oil in cooking and on green salads—so that your diet contains equal amounts of animal fat and vegetable oil. Remember, however, that both fats and oils are high in calories, and there is some evidence to indicate that fat or oil of any kind speeds the aging process and contributes to the development of cancer. For this reason, it's necessary to reduce your intake of fats and oils to prevent the development of disease as well as to prevent a build-up of body fat.

SPECIAL FAT-CONTROL SUPPLEMENTS

A Vitamin E supplement added to your diet will help prevent harmful oxidation of the fatty acids in your body. Be sure to use a natural Vitamin E in the form of capsules containing oil. "Mixed tocopherols" are best. About 200 units for women and 300 units for men will be adequate. Purchase capsules containing 200 units or less so that you can divide your daily intake into three or more doses, preferably before meals and at bedtime.

Supplementing your diet with desiccated liver, lecithin, wheat germ, and brewer's yeast will provide important B vitamins that help combat a build-up of hard fat in your arteries. Vitamin E, Vitamin B_6 (pyridoxine), choline, and inositol are helpful in combating formations of blood fat. Adding a little vegetable oil to your diet will supply essential fatty acids that soften hard fat and aid absorption of fat-soluble vitamins.

You can learn more about how to eat to protect your arteries by reading my book *Doctor Homola's Life-Extender Health Guide* (Parker Publishing Company).

REMEMBER THESE IMPORTANT POINTS

It's well known that *refined carbohydrate in the diet is the biggest cause of overweight.* Simply substituting *natural* carbohydrate for refined carbohydrate, reducing the amount of fat and carbohydrate in your diet, and eating low-fat protein foods will protect your health as well as prevent a build-up of body fat. Eat chicken and fish as often as possible. Depend upon fruits and vegetables for your carbohydrate. Include a small amount of vegetable oil in your diet for essential fatty acids and fat-soluble vitamins. Don't cook with vegetable oil, however, unless absolutely necessary. Instead, use a tablespoonful of cold-pressed vegetable oil daily on a tossed salad. (Wheat germ oil is rich in Vitamin E and essential fatty acids. Safflower oil is a good source of the essential fatty acids, but it does not contain much Vitamin

E. If you use oils other than wheat germ oil, it might be a gooa idea to take a Vitamin E supplement to prevent oxidation of the fatty acids.)

Nicotine and Caffeine Raise Blood Fat

Cigarettes and coffee contain powerful stimulants that may raise blood fat by stimulating the adrenal glands. This may result in a pancreatic reaction that removes sugar from the blood for storage as fat. So don't get into the habit of drinking coffee or tea between meals, even if it is unsweetened.

HOW THE BASIC NATURAL FOODS IMPROVE HEALTH AND DISINTEGRATE FAT

Everyone is familiar with the seven basic food groups that nutritionists recommend for good health. These same seven food groups should form the core of your reducing diet—with a few special variations. Remember that any type of diet you go on to lose weight must not damage your health. If you eat at least one food from each of the seven basic food groups each day, you'll be assured of getting adequate nutrients. And if you select fresh, *naturai* foods rather than canned, frozen, or packaged foods, you'll have a better chance of getting the 40 or more nutrients that are known to be essential for good health. There are undoubtedly many more essential nutrients that have not yet been discovered. In order to get *all* of the known and unknown nutrients, it's absolutely necessary to develop your diet around the seven basic food groups. Your body must be metabolically balanced in order for it to dispose of excess fat and normalize its weight, and this requires *balanced* nutrition.

Many overweight people are actually undernourished. An excessive amount of body fat is usually associated with unbalanced eating that results in poor health or nutritional deficiency. Whether you are overweight or not, you should eat some of all the basic foods in order to fight fat, but not too much of the type of food that forms fat.

Basically, there are three types of foods: protein, carbohydrate, and fat. Protein is found in such foods as meat, fish, poultry, milk, cheese, eggs, beans, seeds, and grains. Carbohydrate is supplied by fruits, vegetables, and grains. Animal products are the richest sources of fat. On my diet, you'll be reducing your intake of animal fat and substituting a small amount of vegetable oil. Natural carbohydrates are not nearly as fattening as refined carbohydrates, but it might be necessary to reduce your intake of certain high-carbohydrate natural foods. You'll learn in Chapter 3 how to go on a specific reducing diet. First, however, you must learn something about the seven basic food groups.

The Seven Basic Food Groups in Everyday Eating

The seven basic food groups you'll be using on my fat-disintegrator diet are as follows:

(1) Green and yellow vegetables

(2) Citrus fruit, tomatoes, and raw cabbage

(3) Potatoes and other vegetables and fruits

(4) Skimmed milk and skimmed milk products, such as cottage cheese and yogurt

(5) Lean meat, skinned poultry, fish, eggs, and dried peas and beans

(6) Whole-grain bread, cereals, and flour

(7) Vegetable oil and Vitamin E

The reason you must select one food from each group in balancing your diet is that each food group supplies certain essential nutrients. Fruits and vegetables, for example, supply Vitamin C and natural carbohydrate. Green and yellow vegetables supply Vitamin A. Vegetables also supply a certain amount of calcium, but you must include milk products to make sure that you get all the calcium you need for strong bones and healthy teeth. Lean meats supply B vitamins and iron along with protein for building body tissue. Ocean fish should be eaten as often as possible, since it is low in fat and rich in the iodine you need for a healthy thyroid gland. Remember that thyroid trouble caused by an iodine deficiency can make it difficult or impossible to control your bodyweight. Whole-grain breads and cereals supply the Vitamin E you must have for healthy blood vessels and a strong heart.

There are, of course, many other nutrients your body must have to be strong and healthy. You can get all of them in adequate amounts if you plan your diet around the seven basic food groups. You can do so and still reduce your bodyweight if you observe the rules outlined in this book.

SPECIAL SUPPLEMENTS FOR A LOW-FAT DIET

Since Vitamins A and D are fat soluble and tend to be deficient in a diet that reduces your intake of animal fat, it might be a good idea to take a supplement containing these vitamins. Remember, however, that excessive amounts of any fat-soluble vitamin can have harmful effects, so you should not take large doses over a long period of time. The minimum daily requirement for Vitamin A is usually given as 5,000 units, and that of Vitamin D as 400 units. I usually recommend up to 15,000 units of Vitamin A and 1,000 units of Vitamin D daily. You can also get Vitamin D from sunlight and from Vitamin D enriched milk. The carotene in green and yellow vegetables can be converted into Vitamin A in your body.

Vitamin E is also a fat-soluble vitamin. If you eat fresh vegetables and whole-grain products every day, you'll probably get all the Vitamin E you need. But since you'll be substituting vegetable oil for animal fat on my fat-disintegrator diet, I would recommend that you take a few hundred units of Vitamin E each day to protect the essential fatty acids supplied by the oil.

A SPECIAL NOTE FOR VEGETARIANS

If you are knowledgeable about the amino acid content of the various vegetables, you might be able to combine certain vegetables to form a complete protein that can be used by your body to rebuild tissue. Remember, however, that the Vitamin B$_{12}$ you need to prevent the development of anemia is found almost exclusively in foods of animal origin. So if you don't eat meat, you should at least eat eggs, cheese, and milk products along with fish and poultry—or take a Vitamin B$_{12}$ supplement.

HOW TO USE THE BASIC FOODS

In order to simplify selections of foods in your daily diet, I have condensed the seven basic food groups into four groups: the meat group, the vegetable and fruit group, the milk group, and the bread and cereal group.

Meat group. In the meat group, you should eat at least two or more servings each day (three ounces each serving) of beef, veal, lamb, poultry, fish, or eggs. Dry peas and beans also supply protein, but since they are fairly high in carbohydrate you should go easy on them until you have reduced your bodyweight to where you want it. Seeds and nuts contain a nearly complete protein, but they are fairly high in fat.

Chicken and fish are the best sources of low-fat protein. They do not contain the hidden fat found in beef. And the fat they do contain is largely unsaturated, which means that it won't harden in your arteries. If you bake or broil your chicken and fish, you can eat as much as you want without fear of increasing your body fat or damaging your health. In fact, if you eat *large* servings of chicken and fish four or five days a week, you'll be less inclined to eat too much of other types of foods, especially carbohydrates that contribute fattening calories. It's important, however, that you eat some of all the basic foods in order to balance your diet and to assure adequate nutrition.

Vegetable and fruit group. You should have at least four one-half-cup servings daily of vegetables and fruits. This should include a citrus fruit (orange or grapefruit) or some other fruit or vegetable that is rich in Vitamin C, such as cantaloupe, fresh strawberries, broccoli, or green peppers. Other vegetables to choose from, all of which contain some Vitamin C, include asparagus tips, brussels sprouts, raw cabbage, collards, garden cress, kale, kohlrabi, mustard greens, potatoes and sweet potatoes cooked in their jacket, spinach, rutabagas, tomatoes and tomato juice, and turnip greens.

Other fruits include honeydew melon, tangerines and tangerine juice, lemons and lemon juice, and watermelon.

You should eat at least one dark-green or deep-yellow vegetable every day for the Vitamin A it supplies. You can choose from broccoli, carrots, chard, collards, cress, mustard greens, kale, pumpkin, spinach, sweet potatoes, turnip greens, and other dark-green leafy vegetables, or winter squash. Apricots and cantaloupe also supply Vitamin A.

Fresh green salads with plenty of tomatoes, lettuce, and raw cabbage will provide filling bulk as well as Vitamin C. Remember that you need all the cellulose you can get to keep your bowels clean and healthy. A large salad before a main meal will provide cellulose as well as take the edge off your appetite. If you lace the salad with a tablespoonful of vegetable oil, such as corn oil, safflower oil, or wheat germ oil, you can get the essential fatty acids you need without eating butter, meat fat, and other types of animal fat.

I do not believe that a moderate amount of any properly prepared natural food is fattening, no matter how many calories it contains. In the early weeks of your diet, however, it might be a good idea to go easy on starchy fruits and vegetables such as peas, beans, corn, potatoes, apples, and bananas. Actually, natural carbohydrates, which usually contain a large amount of indigestible fiber, provide bulk that aids the body's appetite mechanism in telling you when you have had enough to eat. So it's not likely that you'll eat too much of any natural food.

Milk group. Every adult should have two or more cups of *skim milk*—or its equivalent—for bone-building calcium. The lactose in milk, however, commonly causes intestinal discomfort or "indigestion." If you cannot tolerate milk, you can get the calcium you need from fermented milk products. The lactose in buttermilk, cottage cheese, and yogurt, for example, has been converted to lactic acid by bacterial action. Fermented milk products made from *skimmed milk* are low in fat and high in protein.

Between-meal snacks of yogurt and cottage cheese with a little fresh fruit will help reduce your mealtime appetite. Farmer cheese and pot cheese, which are varieties of cottage cheese, are also a good bet for reducing diets. Weight watchers can make a good fat-fighting meal out of cottage cheese and fresh fruit.

Remember that you must fight fat by *eating* to keep your blood sugar level up and to provide nutrients that will prevent an abnormal craving for sweets, fats, and carbohydrates.

Bread and cereal group. You should go easy on bread of any kind when you are on a reducing diet. Four or more servings daily of whole-grain products are usually recommended as part of a balanced diet. One slice of bread, one ounce of ready-to-eat *natural* cereal, or one-half to three-quarters of a cup of cooked cereal represents one serving. (Don't buy "quick cooking" cereals.) Obviously, if you eat cereal you must eat less bread. If you eat no other whole-grain products, you may eat whole-grain bread with each meal. Choose from corn bread, whole wheat, rye, pumpernickel, and such whole-grain cereals as rye, oats, barley, wheat, grits, corn, and brown rice. All types of whole-grain products supply essential bran and Vitamin E. They aren't as fattening as refined bread, cereals, and flour, and they are much more nourishing.

If you must sweeten your cereal, try using raisins. Honey is a nutritious sweetener, but remember that it is just as high in calories as sugar.

Note: Avoid refined bread and cereals as if they were poison. In addition to being high in fattening calories, they are deficient in nutrients and often contain artificial additives.

WHAT ABOUT BEVERAGES?

Be sure to drink plenty of liquids during the day. *Always use water to satisfy your thirst.* You should drink fruit and vegetable juices rather than coffee, tea, soda, or alcohol. Sugar-sweetened beverages and alcohol destroy B vitamins in your body as well as disturb your blood sugar. This can lead to an abnormal craving for food that may make it difficult or impossible to stay on a reducing diet.

Although fruit juices make a good beverage, remember that it's always better to eat the whole fruit than to squeeze it for juice. Fruit pulp helps cut down on calorie intake by providing filling bulk. A good rule to follow is to *eat fruit* and *drink vegetable juice*. Since vegetable juice has fewer calories than fruit juice, *you can drink unlimited amounts of vegetable juices*.

Don't worry about drinking too much water. You can't get fat drinking water. Excessive use of salt, however, may force your body to retain too much water. Use as little salt as possible on your foods. If you're not an athlete or laborer who perspires heavily, you can get all the salt your body needs from natural foods.

Beware of Artificially Sweetened Beverages

I do not recommend the use of artificial sweeteners, since they may have harmful effects on your health. At least one artificial sweetener, for example, has been suspected to be a cause of cancer. There's no point in sacrificing your health in order to lose a few pounds of fat. The type of beverages that require sweetening, such as coffee, tea, and soda pop, usually contain harmful ingredients. You can do without them. If you drink water, juices, skim milk, and other wholesome beverages, you won't need to use sweeteners of any kind.

Note: Although large doses of cyclamates have been shown to cause cancer in rats, no one knows the long-range effects of this artificial sweetener in the foods and beverages of humans. Cyclamates were removed from the market a few years ago. But since it has not been demonstrated that cyclamates can cause cancer in humans, they may soon be returned to the market for limited use. The dangers of cyclamates and other artificial sweeteners may be questionable, but the dangers are a real possibility. So don't use them just because they are available. This is no guarantee that they are safe. They certainly have no nutritional value.

SUMMARY

1. In addition to containing more bulk and fewer calories, natural foods often contain bran, fiber, or cellulose that aids elimination and improves the health of the bowels.

2. Excessive use of sugar and other refined carbohydrates can contribute to the development of overweight and hardened arteries just as surely as excessive use of fat-rich foods.

3. In order to control your bodyweight and protect your health, you'll have to eliminate refined carbohydrates and cut down on animal fat.

4. A little Vitamin E and a small amount of vegetable oil added to your diet will help counteract the harmful effects of fats and oils in your diet.

5. A diet made up of *natural* carbohydrates and low-fat protein foods is the cornerstone of any good health-building, weight-reducing diet.

6. Every reducing diet should contain something from *all* the seven basic food groups in order to insure adequate amounts of all the nutrients known to be essential for good health.

7. Supplements containing Vitamins A and D are often added to a low-fat diet.

8. If you limit food selections to the basic natural foods, your appetite mechanism will automatically control your intake of calories.

9. Use *water* to satisfy your thirst and drink skimmed milk and juices instead of coffee, tea, or soda pops.

10. *The next chapter will tell you how to go on a day-to-day fat-disintegrator diet.*

3

How to Go on
My Fat-Disintegrator Diet
One Week at a Time

If you're not sure whether you are overweight or not, stand nude before a full-length mirror and take a good look at yourself. Is your waist wider than your hips? Are the youthful lines of your body hidden by layers of bulging fat? If the image you see in the mirror appears to be fat, then you can safely assume that you're too fat. If you can pinch-up more than an inch of fat on the back of your upper arm, there's no doubt that you have a little extra weight to lose.

SCALES CAN BE MISLEADING

It's nice to have a pair of scales to weigh yourself occasionally, but you cannot be guided entirely by how much you weigh. The image you see in the mirror is probably the most reliable guide in judging your bodyweight. If you don't look fat, then it's not likely that you're too fat, and it's not important how much you weigh. Some heavily muscled or big-boned persons may be "overweight" without being fat.

Consult the weight chart in this chapter to see how your weight compares with that of the average person your own height. Remember, however, that the mirror and the pinch test may be more revealing tests for excess body fat.

When testing for *loss* of bodyweight, you'll have to weigh yourself on a pair of scales. But don't use them too often. Weight loss is normally very slow. Since bodyweight fluctuates from day to day, weighing yourself daily will prove to be discouraging. If you'll just weigh yourself once a week, you'll be able to see some obvious progress in reducing your bodyweight. A loss of two or more pounds a week will eventually rid you of excess body fat.

Don't Be in too Big of a Hurry

Remember that it's better to lose weight slowly than to lose several pounds a week. The type of diet that results in a slow but progressive loss of *excess* body fat is likely to be a sensible diet that will allow your bodyweight to normalize itself. You can stay on such a diet for the rest of your life without making any additional or drastic changes in your eating habits.

How Morgan T. Normalized His Bodyweight

I placed Morgan T. on a "reducing diet" that consisted of nothing more than a few basic rules—such as those outlined in Chapter 2. He lost 30 pounds of excess weight in two months. When I saw him a year later, he was still eating by the same rules. But since he had lost all of his excess body fat many months earlier, he was no longer losing weight. *The same diet that had gotten rid of his excess body fat was maintaining a lean and healthy body.* Morgan did not find it necessary to make any further changes in his eating habits.

"I like the way I'm eating," he said. "And I like the natural foods in my diet. I can now eat all I want without losing *or* gaining. What more could you ask for?"

If you are following the general dietary guides outlined in Chapters 1 and 2, you may already be doing all you need to do to lose weight. If you feel that weight loss is too slow, however, you may need some additional guidance. The material in the remaining portion of this chapter is an important step toward more effective weight reduction.

Check your weight on the following weight chart to see how you compare with others of your height. Then weigh yourself and record the weight for comparison in the weeks to come.

WEIGHT CHART FOR MEN

Height (in shoes)	Small Frame	Medium Frame	Large Frame
5'2"	112-120	118-129	126-141
3"	115-123	121-133	129-144
4"	118-126	124-136	132-148
5"	121-129	127-139	135-152
6"	124-133	130-143	138-156
7"	128-137	134-147	142-161
8"	132-141	138-152	147-166
9"	136-145	142-156	151-170
10"	140-150	146-160	155-174
11"	144-154	150-165	159-179
6'0"	148-158	154-170	164-184
1"	152-162	158-175	168-189
2"	156-167	162-180	173-194
3"	160-171	167-185	178-199
4"	164-175	172-190	182-204

WEIGHT CHART FOR WOMEN

Height (in shoes)	Small Frame	Medium Frame	Large Frame
4'10"	92- 98	96-107	104-119
11"	94-101	98-110	106-122
5'0"	96-104	101-113	109-125
1"	99-107	104-115	112-128
2"	102-110	107-119	115-131
3"	105-113	110-122	118-134
4"	108-116	113-126	121-138
5"	111-119	116-130	125-142
6"	114-123	120-135	129-146
7"	118-127	124-139	133-150
8"	122-131	128-143	137-154
9"	126-135	132-147	141-158
10"	130-140	136-151	145-163
11"	134-144	140-155	149-168
6'0"	138-148	144-159	153-173

IMPORTANT BASIC RULES FOR REDUCING FAT

In order to refresh your memory and to emphasize certain important points, some of the suggestions offered in Chapter 1 will be repeated in this chapter. Instructions will be more detailed, however, since you'll be following a stricter set of rules. But don't worry. You won't be required to follow a specific diet, and you'll be allowed to select the foods you want to eat. As I said earlier, my "diet" is not really a diet; it is a *guide*. Nevertheless, it has proved to be more effective than the type of diet that tells you exactly what to eat at every meal.

The First Rule of Successful Reducing: Eliminate Processed Foods!

When you stop eating processed foods and refined carbohydrates, chances are your body will immediately begin burning some of its stored fat for energy. Remember that sugar and refined carbohydrates flood the blood with glucose, resulting in a pancreatic reaction that stores excessive amounts of blood sugar as fat. This causes the individual to *crave* sweets. So be sure to *abstain completely from refined carbohydrates and sweets*. You'll get all the carbohydrate you need from fresh fruits and vegetables.

An overweight school teacher who had a habit of nibbling on refined snacks solved her weight problem simply by eliminating the snacks and eating nothing but fresh, natural foods. "I always thought that reducing was difficult and painful," she confessed. "If I had known ten years ago what I know now, I never would have gotten fat."

You don't have to be burdened with excess body fat because of ignorance. You can lose fat or avoid getting fat simply by following the same basic rules I outline for all my patients. Eliminating refined and processed foods is the most important single step you can take to reduce your bodyweight.

You Must Eat to Reduce Safely

Don't ever let anyone tell you that you must starve yourself to lose weight. Actually, it's best to eat regularly to avoid the fluctuating blood sugar that results in an uncontrollable appetite. It might even be good idea to snack between meals so that you won't have a big appetite at mealtime. Fresh fruit, cottage cheese, tuna packed in water, baked chicken, boiled eggs, raw vegetables, yogurt, or some other low-fat snack will help curb your appetite. Eat *small* snacks, and then be careful not to stuff yourself during regular meals. If you eat strictly natural foods that have not been seasoned with condiments, gravy, and other appetite stimulants, it's not likely that you'll overeat. In fact, chances are you'll eat *less* in six meals than you normally would in three meals.

Persons who eat big meals once or twice a day may become fat simply because they flood their blood with more sugar and fat than they can possibly use immediately. The excess is then quickly stored as body fat in order to balance the contents of the blood. This won't happen when the body is fed several times a day in small amounts.

You'll Get All the Fat You Need from Lean Meats

Although my fat-disintegrator diet is low in fat, it contains all the fat you need for good health. Lean meats, for example, contain a considerable amount of invisible fat. Just to make sure that you do not get too much fat, you should cut away all the visible fat before cooking meat. Beef, veal, and lamb are not as fat as pork, so avoid pork whenever possible. Veal is lowest in fat.

Chicken and fish have fewer calories and less hard fat than any of the meats. You can eat all the chicken and fish you want if they are not fried or cooked in oil or gravy.

Note: *Do not eat processed meats*, no matter how lean they may appear to be. Many processed lunch meats contain sugar, additives, and other harmful ingredients.

Keep Potatoes Simple

Potatoes are among nature's richest sources of carbohydrate. You need carbohydrate for energy, but too much carbohydrate supplies calories that are easily converted to fat.

So while you should include potatoes in a balanced diet, you should probably eat less of them than other vegetables. If you bake or boil your potatoes, it's not likely that you'll eat too many. Your appetite mechanism will let you know when you have had enough. You should avoid french fries, scalloped potatoes, buttered or mashed potatoes, and other tasty potato dishes that have been made more appetizing with special cooking methods. Your appetite mechanism won't have a chance if it is stimulated with fancy cooking.

When you eat a baked potato, *always eat the jacket,* since it contains important nutrients and roughage. Make sure that your cook *washes* the potato before cooking, however, so that you won't bite down on sand or grit. I once advised a friend of mine to eat the potato jacket when we were served a steak and potato in a fancy restaurant. He promptly bit into a small rock! I'm sure that most restaurants wash their potatoes before baking them. I *always* eat the whole potato, and I have never bitten into sand or grit.

MOST VEGETABLES ARE LOW IN CARBOHYDRATE

When you want extra helpings of vegetables, select *leafy* vegetables. They contain more bulk in the form of indigestible cellulose. They also contain less carbohydrate. Some vegetables are, of course, rich in carbohydrate. So you'll have to be selective in what you eat.

Low-Carbohydrate Vegetables

There are a number of low-carbohydrate vegetables to choose from in planning your meals. Vegetables that contain only three to six percent carbohydrate, for example, are asparagus, broccoli, celery, brussels sprouts, cabbage, cauliflower, cucumber, eggplant, endive, lettuce, mustard greens (and greens of all kinds), green pepper, okra, radish, sauerkraut, sorrel, spinach, string beans, summer squash, tomatoes, watercress, zucchini, artichokes, beets, carrots, celeriac, dandelion greens, kale, kohlrabi, leeks, onions, parsley, young peas, pumpkin, rutabaga, and turnips.

With such a variety of vegetables to choose from, you can eat something different every day. If you're not anxious to lose more than a couple of pounds a week, you can eat generously of all these vegetables. Properly prepared, fresh vegetables can be tasty as well as nourishing.

High-Carbohydrate Vegetables

Fortunately, there are only a few high-carbohydrate vegetables that must be restricted in a weight-reducing diet. Peas, beans, corn, and potatoes, for example, are about 15 to 20 percent carbohydrate. This means that you may have to eat them sparingly—depending upon whether you are losing or gaining weight.

If your diet is strictly limited to *natural* foods, you may be able to lose two or more pounds a week no matter what type of vegetables you eat. But if weight loss is slow or nonexistent, you may have to reduce or eliminate the high-carbohydrate vegetables—or take regular exercise. (Persons who are active or who take regular exercise can usually eat generously of any natural food without gaining weight.)

BE GUIDED BY COMMON SENSE

Common sense should be your guide in following my fat-disintegrator diet. A little trial and error based on a knowledge of foods will enable you to adjust your diet according to gains or losses in bodyweight.

You'll learn in Chapter 4 how to prepare vegetables for maximum nutrition and minimum calories. In the meantime, just remember to eat your vegetables *plain*. A little salt and pepper is all the seasoning you need.

FRUITS SHOULD BE A PART OF YOUR REDUCING DIET

Most fruits contain sugar and carbohydrate. It's not likely, however, that you'll eat an excessive amount of any kind of fruit—provided it's *fresh* fruit and not canned fruit. I have never heard of anyone getting fat by eating too much fresh fruit. Bananas and apples are fairly rich in carbohydrate, but few people ever eat more than one serving of either of these fruits. I personally find it difficult to eat more than one apple. A single banana can curb your appetite. You can usually depend upon your appetite mechanism to control your intake of any type of fresh fruit, and you can use fresh fruit to reduce your appetite for more fattening foods.

Dried fruits are so rich in sugar that they should be eaten sparingly until your weight is down where you want it. When a fruit has been dried, loss of water reduces the fruit to a smaller size, concentrating the sugar into a calorie-rich sweet. Such concentrated carbohydrate might stimulate your appetite if you have a sweet tooth, so you may have to avoid eating much dried fruit. Many people find that cheese and fresh fruit can be substituted for sweet desserts after meals. (Cheese and fresh fruit combined are a popular "dessert" in France.) If fresh fruits do not satisfy your sweet tooth and you *must* have something sweet, eat a little dried fruit following a noon or evening meal.

Note: Most fruits contain less than one percent fat, with the exception of avocados and olives, which are rich in fat.

HAVE A WHOLE-GRAIN PRODUCT
AT LEAST ONCE DAILY

Whole-grain products are fairly high in carbohydrate, but they should be a part of every balanced diet. A whole-grain cereal for breakfast, for example, or a few slices of whole-grain bread or corn bread each day will supply important bran as well as essential nutrients. Just be careful not to eat too much bread. If you have cereal for breakfast, you don't need toast. You can, however, have one slice of pure whole-grain bread with noon and evening meals. If you snack between meals, do not eat sandwiches made with bread. If you must have a "sandwich," use lettuce leaves instead of bread. Peanut butter and other natural spreads can be smeared over slices of fruit.

Most grocery stores stock a variety of whole-grain breads and cereals. Wheat germ, whole wheat, barley, oat groats, rye, bran flakes, grits, oats, long-grain brown rice, and mixed natural cereals are now readily available. Whole-grain bread that does not contain preservatives and other additives can often be found in coolers along with other perishable products.

Note: Always purchase old-fashioned grits or oatmeal. The quick-cooking variety may be deficient in fiber.

USE SKIMMED MILK PRODUCTS

Milk products are essential in any diet, since they provide calcium that strengthens bones and protects teeth. In order to protect your arteries and reduce the amount of fat in your diet, however, you should drink skimmed milk—or use skimmed milk products. A glass of skimmed milk has only half the calories found in a glass of whole milk. Cottage cheese, farmer cheese, pot cheese, and yogurt are good fat-fighting foods when made from skimmed milk.

Even when made from whole milk, yogurt has been found to be effective in lowering blood cholesterol. But it's always best to make yogurt from skimmed milk to reduce its calorie content. Lactobacillus acidophilus is the best culture to use for improved intestinal health. (See Chapter 4 for instructions in preparing yogurt at home.)

FILL UP WITH GREEN SALADS

Fresh, raw salads should also be a part of your reducing diet. In fact, you should make a special effort to precede your noon and evening meals with a large bowl of salad. This will reduce your appetite for more fattening foods as well as supply moisture-retaining cellulose that helps prevent constipation, diverticulitis, colon cancer, and other intestinal disorders.

Regardless of what you eat, always stop eating when you are comfortably full. If a salad fills you up, don't stuff yourself in order to eat some of all the basic foods. What you don't eat today, you can eat tomorrow. You'll learn later in this chapter how to alternate the basic food groups in order to reduce the quantity of food you eat.

You can put any type of edible, raw vegetable into your salads—and the more variety the better. In addition to lettuce and tomatoes, for example, you can add carrots, sprouts, diced sweet potatoes, cabbage, celery, cucumbers, onions, radishes, raw stalks of broccoli, raw cauliflower flowerets, green peppers, and cooked string beans and beets. A small amount of salt with vinegar and lemon juice will make a good low-fat dressing. It might also be a good idea to include a tablespoonful of vegetable oil—preferably Vitamin E-rich wheat germ oil—for essential fatty acids.

If green salads form gas in your intestines, eat your salads in the evening so that you won't be bothered during the day with gas pains.

When you eat a salad containing a variety of fresh, raw vegetables, you don't need to eat cooked vegetables. And if you want to make a *complete* meal of salad, add tuna, chicken, or boiled eggs for protein. With a little imagination, you can make up a tasty salad that contains something from all the seven basic food groups. Remember that on my fat-disintegrator diet, I expect you to use a little common sense in applying what you learn from reading this book. If your diet is limited to fresh, natural foods, your appetite mechanism and your instincts will help you develop the eating habits you need to normalize your bodyweight by disintegrating excess body fat.

THREE SAMPLE MENUS FOR DAILY USE

Just to give you some idea of what you should eat on a balanced weight-reducing diet, I have outlined three sample menus for one day—breakfast, lunch, and dinner. If you follow this general guide each day, you won't have to eat something you don't like or something that's not readily available. All you have to do is select certain basic foods each day, but you must make an effort to select a *different* food in each group as often as possible.

Breakfast

Any whole-grain cereal with skimmed milk (sweetened with raisins or diced fruit if desired) *or* one slice of whole-grain bread.

Eggs *or* lean meat such as ham, Canadian bacon, steak, veal, and so on. Try to have eggs two days a week and lean meat on other days.

One citrus fruit *or* a glass of fruit juice.

Lunch

Lean meat, chicken, or fish—preferably chicken or fish.

One dark-green or deep-yellow vegetable.

One other vegetable of your choice.

One slice of whole-grain bread *or* corn bread.

Skimmed milk, vegetable juice, or water. Remember that vegetable juice has fewer calories than fruit juice. V8 Cocktail Vegetable Juice is a highly nourishing, low-calorie mixture of vegetable juices.

Optional: Melon, fresh fruit, or dried fruit for dessert. You may find that a little unprocessed cheese with fresh fruit is more satisfying than a sweet dessert.

Dinner

Whatever type of meat you have left over from lunch *or* a serving of cottage cheese, pot cheese, or farmer cheese.

One or more servings of leftover vegetables.

A fresh, raw vegetable salad with a vegetable oil dressing.

Skimmed milk or juice.

Optional: A bedtime snack of cottage cheese and fresh fruit—*only if you feel hungry.*

Note: Try to include two glasses of skimmed milk or buttermilk in your daily diet. Fish should be eaten as often as possible, liver at least once a week.

How Andy and Faye Used These Sample Menus

Andy B. took a copy of my sample menus home to his wife, Faye, who pinned it on the kitchen bulletin board. Andy was a sedentary salesman in a men's clothing store and had been steadily gaining weight. Faye spent most of her time at home nibbling on packaged snacks, so she, too, was considerably overweight. Both Andy and Faye were able to lose about three pounds a week by following the general guides of the sample menus. Since both remained fairly inactive, there was no doubt that the diet alone was effective in reducing their bodyweight. After they had each lost 15 or 20 pounds, however, they did become more active, which helped speed the loss of their remaining excess body fat.

"We both look and feel so much better since we've slimmed down," Andy reported, "that we're getting out more and getting more exercise. The diet is great, however, and we intend to stay on it from now on. It's not at all like being on a diet."

You should be able to lose your excess body fat without performing callisthenics, but you should take every opportunity you get to burn a few calories with recreational activity. You'll get a little guidance in this direction in Chapter 7. Even sexual activities, as you'll learn in that chapter, can provide calorie-burning exercise!

LET YOUR APPETITE BE YOUR GUIDE

Some people prefer to eat their main meal at noon, while others eat more at evening meals. Many doctors recommend that you eat a light evening meal to curb overnight storage of calories as fat, and then eat a good breakfast to correct a drop in blood sugar. This goes along with the old saying, "Eat breakfast like a king, dinner like a prince, and supper like a pauper." You should be careful, however, not to eat too much at any meal. An overfilled stomach makes it difficult to think and work, in addition to building up fat stores.

If you follow my suggestions and eat properly, you won't be inclined to overeat at mealtime. Just remember not to stuff yourself. Eat fairly light meals of natural foods. Then, if you feel hungry between meals, you can eat a snack of fresh fruit or some low-fat protein food, such as cottage cheese or baked chicken. Whenever you do eat a between-meal snack, you should eat *less* at mealtime. If you have a bedtime snack, for example, your blood sugar won't be so low in the morning that you must eat a large breakfast.

Be guided by your appetite. Eat when you're hungry, but eat lightly! If you eat strictly natural foods, chances are you'll eat less in six meals than in three. Your appetite mechanism will rarely fail you if you do not include refined or processed foods in your diet.

HOW TO ALTERNATE THE BASIC FOOD GROUPS

It really does not matter what foods you eat at lunch or dinner as long as you eat enough of a variety to cover the recommended food groups. If you find that it's difficult to eat some of all the basic foods every day without stuffing yourself, you may alternate some of them to make sure that you get the variety you need throughout the week. For example, you should eat a dark-green or deep-yellow vegetable at least every-other-day. You may then eat a different vegetable on alternate days. If you have a vegetable with your noon and evening meal and have fruit at breakfast and in the evening, you'll have the recommended four servings daily of the fruit and vegetable group. A fresh, green salad can, of course, serve as a vegetable. (Turn back to Chapter 2 and review the material on how to use the basic food groups.)

It's always a good idea to have protein-rich meat, fish, poultry, or eggs in at least two meals each day. But on days when you don't have flesh foods or eggs, you can have milk products (preferably cottage cheese, pot cheese, or farmer cheese) or dried peas or beans (preferably soybeans). Nuts and nut butters also contain protein, but remember that they are rich in fat. Peas and beans, with the exception of soybeans, are rich in carbohydrate. So whenever possible, it's best to get your protein from chicken, fish, or cottage cheese.

In the bread and cereal group, you can have whole-grain cereal *or* bread for breakfast. You don't need them both in the same meal. If you have corn bread with noon and evening meals, you don't need any other form of bread during the day. On days when you do have corn bread, eat green, leafy vegetables rather than starchy vegetables so that you won't have an excessive amount of carbohydrate. The southern dish of "corn bread and collard greens" is a good example of a healthful and tasty combination of foods.

Good dieting is just good, common sense. If you eat a variety of *natural* foods, making sure that you *cover the four basic food groups over a period of at least two days,* you can eat less and still get adequate nutrition.

COOK ONCE EACH DAY

When you cook at home, *always plan your daily meals so that you will have enough food left over from your noon meal to serve at your evening meal.* It's an unnecessary expense to prepare two different meals for lunch and dinner. *It's never a good idea, however, to prepare more food than you can eat in one day.* Food left over from one day to the next loses nutrients (but retains calories) and is therefore less healthful and more fattening than freshly prepared foods. Remember that when you become nutritionally deficient, you crave more food, usually sweets and carbohydrates.

Vitamin Supplements for Nutritional Insurance

When you find it difficult or impossible to eat some of *all* the basic foods over a two-day period, you should take a good multiple vitamin supplement, even if you are not on a diet.

If you find it necessary to greatly reduce servings of the basic foods in order to lose weight, you should take a vitamin-mineral supplement just to be safe. Remember, however, that natural foods contain undiscovered elements that may be just as essential to good health as the known vitamins and minerals. So be sure to *depend first upon natural foods for your vitamins and minerals*—and then use supplements as a form of nutritional insurance.

HOW TO CUT DOWN ON CALORIES WITHOUT COUNTING CALORIES

I have not stressed counting calories for the simple reason that few people can continue a calorie-counting diet for very long. Furthermore, it has been my experience that dieting is much more successful in the long run if food selections are limited to fresh, natural foods that have been properly prepared. This will automatically limit the number of calories in your diet—and the calories you do take in won't be as fattening as those found in processed foods. The calories in natural foods are not so easily absorbed. An increased amount of indigestible fiber supplied by natural foods may actually *hinder* intestinal absorption of calories (see Chapter 4). Natural foods also supply bulk that fills the stomach with low-calorie food. So even if you don't count calories on my natural foods diet, you are limiting your intake of calories by substituting natural foods for processed foods.

If you find weight loss too slow after a few months on an unlimited diet of natural foods, you can cut calories even further by cutting down on the quantity of food you eat.

A Simple Formula for Counting Calories

If you'd like to try a calorie-counting diet, there is a simple formula that you can use to determine how many calories your meals must contain for you to lose weight.

It's well known that there are 3,500 calories in one pound of body fat. This means that if you take in 1,000 less calories per day than you need to maintain your *existing* bodyweight, you can *lose* two pounds a week. It takes about 12 to 15 calories per pound of bodyweight to *maintain* your bodyweight—12 for women and 15 for men. If you are a man and you weigh 200 pounds, for example, you would need 3,000 calories daily (15 x

200= 3,000) to keep from losing weight. Reducing your calorie intake to 2,000 calories a day would result in a loss of two pounds a week.

When your weight is down close to where you want it, you may have to *increase* your intake of calories in order to prevent further loss of weight. When you get your weight down to 175 pounds, for example, you can maintain that weight with 2,625 calories daily (175 x 15= 2,625). It may be necessary to keep refiguring your calorie needs as you lose weight so that you won't lose all of your fat reserves or develop a nutritional deficiency.

The calorie-counting method of dieting is largely a hit-and-miss proposition. No one eats exactly the same every day, and it's difficult or impossible to be sure of the calorie content of foods, no matter how they're listed on calorie charts.* (There are many *hidden* calories in processed foods.) If you have developed a pancreatic sensitivity to processed foods or refined carbohydrates, even a small amount of such food can destroy the effectiveness of a low-calorie diet. I have found that if refined foods are *completely eliminated* from the diet, you can take in more calories without gaining weight.

Even on a natural foods reducing diet, you should make an effort to *reduce your intake of high-calorie foods,* such as fats, oils, and concentrated carbohydrates. Since most of the excess calories in the diet of the average American come from *refined* carbohydrates, most people can lose weight simply by cutting down on carbohydrate. Every reducing diet should contain some carbohydrate, however. When there is not enough natural carbohydrate in the diet to supply a portion of the body's energy needs, a rapid weight loss caused by excessive burning of body fat may result in harmful side effects. This is one reason why most doctors recommend that you not lose more than two or three pounds of body fat a week. Reducing is a little slower this way, but it's safer and more permanent.

Fortunately, you can get all the carbohydrate you need from fresh fruits and vegetables.

---

*Many drug stores and newsstands sell calorie-counting booklets that list the calorie content of foods according to size and number of servings.

A STANDARD LOW-CALORIE DIET

Here's an example of a balanced diet that provides about 1,200 calories daily:

Skim milk—2 cups (1 pint), 160 calories

Egg—1 medium, 81 calories

Lean meat, fish, or fowl—4 ounces (cooked), 376 calories

Vegetables (except potatoes)—4 servings (one-half cup each), 140 calories

Fruit, citrus—1 serving
     other fruits—2 servings
     213 calories

Whole-grain bread—2 slices, 135 calories

Butter, margarine, or vegetable oil—1 tablespoonful (3 teaspoons), 100 calories

You can use this diet as a foundation and then add fresh salads, broiled fish, cottage cheese, and other fresh foods as needed, depending upon whether you're losing or gaining weight. If you stick strictly to fresh, *natural* foods, you should be able to take in *more* than 1,200 calories and still lose weight. It's never safe to take in less than 1,200 calories a day if you want to be assured of getting adequate protein, vitamins, and minerals. Some nutritionists maintain that diets that supply fewer than 2,100 to 2,400 calories a day (depending upon bodyweight) are likely to be deficient in nutrients known to be essential for good health. So you probably should not stay on a low-calorie diet for very long, even if you take supplements. It would be better to take exercise so that you can eat more.

If you fail to lose weight fast enough on a 1,200 calorie diet and you want to go on a "crash diet" (Heaven forbid!), you can use the 1,200 calorie diet as a guide and then make these changes: reduce servings of vegetables to one serving of deep green or yellow vegetable, continue to eat one serving of citrus fruit and reduce other fruits to only one serving, omit all bread, and increase servings of meat, fish, or chicken from four ounces to seven ounces. This will reduce the carbohydrate content of the diet to approximately 60 grams and increase your intake of iron and B vitamins. It's absolutely essential, however, that you take a good multiple vitamin-mineral supplement, and then gradually work your way back to a more normal diet after a couple of weeks.

HOW TO PREVENT SIDE EFFECTS
BY CONTROLLING CARBOHYDRATE

Nutritionists estimate that the average adult needs about 100 grams of carbohydrate a day. This is often reduced to 60 grams on a reducing diet. Weight loss may be a little slower when the diet includes at least 60 grams of *natural* carbohydrate, but it will be more permanent. Without adequate carbohydrate in the diet, metabolism of fat may have toxic effects or result in dehydration.

When your body is forced to burn large amounts of stored fat for energy, fatty acid waste products called ketone bodies may begin to appear in your urine. You can test for the presence of these products with Ketostix, a paper strip that changes color when dipped into urine. Ketone bodies may appear in the urine during a high-fat diet; but when they appear during a low-fat, low-carbohydrate diet, it may mean that there is not adequate carbohydrate in the diet. So if ketones begin to appear in your urine, you should stop cutting down on your carbohydrate. The trick is to cut down on your carbohydrates just enough to divide your energy needs between dietary carbohydrate and stored body fat. This will prevent the development of gout, ketosis, and other harmful side effects of a too-rapid weight loss. This is another reason why you should be satisfied with losing only two or three pounds a week. With a properly balanced diet, you will eventually lose *all* of your excess body fat. Best of all, your weight will automatically adjust itself to a normal level without you making any drastic changes in your diet.

A DIET IS ONLY A GUIDE

Remember that a menu is only a guide. Very few people can include the exact foods listed on a variety of different menus for every day of the week. It really does not matter what type of vegetable or meat you eat at mealtime as long as you cover the four basic food groups over a period of two days. You do not have to limit each meal to a certain type of food. If you prefer to eat eggs for dinner, for example, you can do so, and then have steak for breakfast. The important thing is to eat some of all the basic foods over a period of 24 to 48 hours—without stuffing yourself.

GO EASY ON ALCOHOL

If you have a lot of weight to lose, you should, of course, avoid the use of alcohol as a beverage. Your body must dispose of alcohol by burning it in your liver. This supplies energy without nutrients, forcing your body to store food calories as fat. As you learned earlier, the combustion of alcohol in your body will actually *steal* nutrients from your body.

"Dry" whiskey or wine has less sugar than sweet brands, but alcohol itself supplies many calories. Alcohol in the bloodstream may also trigger a pancreatic reaction that *lowers* blood sugar, resulting in a *craving* for alcohol or sweets. So it's not enough to simply avoid "sweet" alcoholic beverages.

If you must have an occasional cocktail, do so as infrequently as possible—and then have only *one*. There's really no reason, however, why you should have to order an alcoholic beverage when you "go out." You can get tomato juice in any lounge or nightclub.

WILL A NATURAL FOODS DIET WORK FOR YOU?

The dietary suggestions outlined in this chapter are so simple that you may wonder if they will work for you. The answer is "Yes, they will!" No matter how little success you may have had with reducing diets in the past, I'm sure that my natural foods reducing diet will prove to be effective in disintegrating your excess body fat and normalizing your bodyweight.

Twenty-six year old Katherine R. was discouraged to the point of tears when she came to see me about her overweight.

"I've tried a number of diets," she confessed, "but they either don't work or I just can't follow them. I simply cannot stay on a 900 calorie diet without suffering the agonies of starvation."

I explained to Katherine that any successful reducing diet must be a lifetime diet. Few people can succeed with a diet that punishes them with hunger. I outlined my natural foods diet for Katherine and instructed her to eat as much as she needed to satisfy her hunger. I gave her this additional advice: "You must completely eliminate all refined and processed foods, and you must not eat anything containing sugar or white flour."

Katherine lost 40 pounds of excess body fat in six months. When she slipped back into dresses that she hadn't been able to wear for several years, she regained her self-confidence and blossomed into a sparkling, happy, and beautiful woman.

The same general dietary measures that worked for Katherine will work for you! You cannot go wrong when you are guided by the laws of nature. If you are truly interested in losing weight, the elimination of refined and processed foods (sugar and flour) will be a small price to pay for a lean body that can be maintained with a generous supply of fresh, natural foods.

How you prepare the foods you eat can be just as important as the type of foods you select. So be sure to study the next chapter carefully.

SUMMARY

1. If the image you see in the mirror appears fat, then you *are* fat!

2. Eliminating refined and processed foods and eating *natural* foods will allow you to eat generously without gaining weight.

3. Fish, skinned chicken, and uncreamed cottage cheese are good sources of low-fat protein.

4. Potatoes can be eaten along with other vegetables if the potatoes are baked in their jacket.

5. Peas, beans, corn, and potatoes are the only vegetables that may have to be eaten sparingly.

6. Fresh fruits should be a part of everyone's diet and may be used to replace sweet desserts.

7. Whole-grain cereals, skimmed milk products, and green salads are essential in a balanced diet, but may be alternated with whole-grain bread, chicken or fish, and vegetables.

8. If you cover all the basic food groups over a period of *two days,* it's not likely that you'll be nutritionally deficient.

9. The sample menus outlined in this chapter are simply guides in selecting the *types* of foods you should eat each day.

10. Depend first upon the basic natural foods for your vitamins and minerals, and then use supplements as nutritional insurance.

4

How to Prepare
Fat-Disintegrating Foods at Home

After you have carefully selected the foods you need to prepare a fat-disintegrating meal, it's very important to prepare them properly. In this chapter, you'll learn how to cook or prepare the basic natural foods so that they will retain the nutrients your body needs to prevent an abnormal craving for food and an unhealthy build-up of body fat. Remember that a balanced diet that supplies *all* the essential nutrients is important in reducing safely and effectively. The dishes you prepare should be plain and simple. You shouldn't use cooking methods that artificially stimulate your appetite. When you are really hungry, simple natural foods will have a delicious taste And if they are properly prepared, your appetite mechanism will let you know when you have had enough to eat.

DON'T FOOL YOURSELF

One of my patients, Ann T., insisted that she ate only natural foods and still had a weight problem. "I prepare balanced meals every day," she said, "and my husband and I both are 30 pounds overweight."

I questioned Ann about how she prepared her foods and learned that she often "dressed up" her vegetables. Asparagus, string beans, and other low-calorie vegetables, for example, were frequently prepared in casseroles that contained flour, processed cheese sauce, bread crumbs, sugar, oil, meat fat, and other high-calorie additives. All Ann had to do to start losing weight was to switch to a simple method of preparing her vegetables. Using the type of cooking methods described in this chapter, both Ann and her husband began losing a couple of pounds a week. "With this new way of cooking," she said, "we don't eat as much as we did before, but we're perfectly satisfied. And since we've started eating less, we feel more like getting out. We've even joined a square dance club!"

EAT FRUITS AND VEGETABLES RAW WHENEVER POSSIBLE

Fruits should always be eaten raw for maximum nutritional value. Many vegetables may also be eaten raw. Some vegetables, however, yield more nutrients when they are cooked. You can get more Vitamin A from a cooked carrot, for example, than from a raw carrot. The reason for this is that cooking softens the tough cellulose that encases the vitamins.

Many vegetables are just as tasty as they are nourishing when eaten raw. Tomatoes, celery, lettuce, carrots, cucumbers, onions, radishes, and cabbage, for example, are commonly eaten raw. Many other vegetables, such as sweet potatoes, turnip roots, and kohlrabi, are edible when raw.

How to Put Variety in Raw Salads

Before you cook any vegetable that can be eaten raw, put aside a small amount for use in a raw salad. Remember that raw vegetable salads supply important low-calorie bulk as well as fat-disintegrating nutrients. Salads should be an important part of any reducing diet.

Here are a few salad combinations you can use for variety:

Grated carrots, diced celery, and cucumber slices.

Spinach, endive or lettuce, with tomato wedges.

Sliced raw cauliflower flowerets, lettuce, chopped green pepper, celery, and pimiento.

Shredded cabbage, cucumber cubes, and slices of celery.

Cooked red kidney beans, thinly sliced celery, and sweet onions.

Cooked cut green beans, crisp bacon bits, sweet pickles, and onion rings.

You can make your own "chef's salad" by mixing together a great variety of cooked and raw vegetables. A mixture of vegetable oil, vinegar, and lemon juice can be used as a dressing.

Always wash salad greens under cold running water and then allow them to drain before adding salad oil. Salads should always be cold and crisp, and the oil should be evenly distributed throughout the salad. Wait until mealtime to begin preparing a salad. Then wait until it is time to *serve* the salad before mixing in the oil.

Note: It's best to *tear* leaves of lettuce and other greens. Leaves that are cut or shredded lose precious juices.

A Low-Calorie Salad Dressing

If you don't want to use an oily dressing on your salad, you can try my favorite tomato-juice dressing. Remember, however, that a small amount of vegetable oil in your diet, preferably on a green salad, will supply the essential fatty acids your body needs to dissolve the hard fat in your tissues. So if you cannot tolerate a little oil on your salad, you should find some other way to use about two tablespoons of vegetable oil daily.

Here is the recipe for a tomato-juice dressing:

Three-quarters of a cup of chilled tomato juice
Two tablespoons of lemon juice or vinegar
Two tablespoons of instant minced onion
One tablespoon of crumbled basil leaves
One-half teaspoon of salt
One-quarter teaspoon of garlic powder
One-eighth teaspoon of lemon-pepper seasoning
Shake well and store in a refrigerator

You can, of course, use your own imagination in making up a salad dressing. Or you may simply use a little salt and nothing else.

HOW TO COOK VEGETABLES FOR BETTER HEALTH AND A LEANER BODY

Just about everyone overcooks vegetables. When a vegetable has been cut and exposed to heat, light, air, and water, it loses vitamins. This loss can be kept to a minimum with proper cooking procedures, however, so that the ratio of nutrients to bulk remains high. Potatoes, for example, should always be baked in their jackets—and the jackets eaten—so that no nutrients are lost.

How to Get the Most Out of a Potato

Select a medium-size potato that weighs about three ounces. Scrub the potato with a vegetable brush in order to clean the skin. Bake for about 50 minutes at 400 degrees Fahrenheit—until the potato is soft enough to penetrate with a fork.

Eat the jacket along with the potato. Remember that the jacket provides filling bulk as well as important nutrients. If some members of your family refuse to eat potato jackets, scoop out the baked potatoes and put the empty shells back in the oven for about five minutes. A potato jacket browned in this manner, seasoned with a little salt, is delicious. The jacket can be served as a vegetable at the next meal. Anyone who enjoys French fries or potato chips will enjoy a browned potato shell.

How to Make Low-Fat Sour Cream

If you like to use sour cream on your baked potatoes, you can make a non-fattening variety from cottage cheese.

Mix two-thirds of a cup of cottage cheese (made from skimmed milk) with one-fourth of a cup of buttermilk. Add one-half teaspoon of lemon juice and mix in a blender. Serve immediately or put in the refrigerator.

More Nutrients from Less Food

Remember that on a fat-disintegrating diet *you need as many nutrients as you can get from smaller amounts of food.* Your body cannot disintegrate fat without certain basic elements, and these are rarely adequate in the type of diet that makes you fat.

All you have to do to lose weight when you first begin dieting is to eliminate sugar and white flour from your diet and stick strictly to natural foods. After you have lost 10 or 15 pounds of excess body fat, however, your body will begin to function more efficiently on fewer calories. This means that you may have to decrease the amount of food you eat in order to continue losing weight. So it's very important to preserve essential food elements with proper cooking methods.

Heat, Light, Water, and Air Destroy Vitamins

Vegetables should always be cooked with as little water as possible for as short a cooking time as possible. If the vegetable must be cut, keep the pieces as large as possible to permit cooking, so that less surface area will be exposed to water and air. When a vegetable is submerged in water, it loses water-soluble vitamins. Air oxidizes certain vitamins. Prolonged or excessive heat destroys heat-sensitive vitamins.

How to Steam Vegetables

Steaming is the best way to cook vegetables. The displacement of oxygen by steam reduces destruction of vitamins, and less heat is required for cooking.

If you have a cooking pot that has a heavy tight-fitting lid, you can use it to steam vegetables with only a small amount of water. Put just enough water in the pot to prevent scorching. Bring the water to a boil and put in the cut vegetables before putting on the lid. Cook with *low heat* until the vegetables are just tender enough to penetrate with a fork. You should never cook a vegetable until it is mushy. Properly cooked, a vegetable should be slightly crisp. (In addition to destroying nutrients, overcooking a vegetable breaks down the cellulose your bowels need to function normally.)

You can also steam vegetables by placing them in a perforated pan that is resting over a pot of boiling water. Make sure that the vegetables are not submerged in the water. The *steam* should do the cooking.

How to Boil Vegetables

When you must boil a vegetable, use this procedure: Put a small amount of water (about one-third the volume of the vegetables you want to cook) into a pot and bring the water to a boil *before* dropping in the vegetables. Cover the pot with a lid and cook just long enough to soften the vegetable.

Frozen vegetables should be dropped into boiling water while they are still frozen. Remember, however, that frozen vegetables are partially cooked during the blanching process that precedes freezing. So they usually require less cooking than raw vegetables.

Note: When you drop vegetables into boiling water, the water may stop boiling due to absorption of heat by the vegetables. You may turn the heat up until the water begins to boil again and then turn the heat down to maintain gentle boiling.

When boiling is completed, use the leftover water as "pot liquor" or soup. Cooking water is loaded with water-soluble vitamins.

Don't Season Your Vegetables with Fat

Whatever method you use to cook your vegetables, do not "season" them with butter, bacon grease, meat fat, or oil. This will only add fat-building, artery-hardening calories. *A small amount of salt is all the seasoning vegetables need.* If you can't use salt because of high blood pressure, and you feel that you must have a seasoning, try using minced parsley, chives, sweet onions, minced celery, green pepper, toasted sesame seeds, horseradish, garlic, celery seeds, sage, and other herbs and spices. Bouillon cubes can be used to flavor vegetables that do not taste good to you.

You can, of course, do without salt and other forms of seasoning. The use of salt in many cases is simply a habit. You can learn to appreciate the taste of vegetables and other foods without depending upon the use of seasoning.

Cook for One Day at a Time

You should never cook more vegetables than you can eat in one day. Leftover vegetables lose nutrients while retaining calories. Remember that your body must have nutrients to dispose of excess fat. Cook just enough vegetables to serve your family through the evening meal. Serve the vegetables as soon after cooking as possible. Keep them covered between meals in order to prevent damaging exposure to air and light.

A Special Rule for Cooking Peas and Beans

All types of peas and beans, with the exception of soybeans, are high in carbohydrate and must be avoided to some extent until you get your weight down. When you do cook dry peas and beans, they must be boiled in a special way in order to conserve nutrients and to get the full benefit of the protein they contain.

First drop the beans into a pot of boiling water and cook them for two minutes. Then remove the pot from the stove and let the beans soak in the cooking water for one hour before finishing the cooking. This will eliminate the customary 15 hours of cold-water soaking. It also permits you to use the soaking water as cooking water, thus retaining all the water-soluble vitamins and minerals.

HOW TO PREPARE LOW-CALORIE
MEAT, CHICKEN, AND FISH

You already know from reading the opening chapters of this book that fish and poultry are best for your arteries, since they are low in saturated fat. They are also low in calories and should be used often in a reducing diet. Fish, for example, contains only about three percent fat compared with about 40 percent in most meats. All types of lean meats, however, especially veal, will fit in your fat-disintegrator diet if they are properly prepared. If you cut away all the visible fat from meat *before* you cook it, you'll eliminate many calories and a lot of fat. When you peel the skin from fish or poultry, you eliminate practically all of the fat. (You might prefer to remove the skin of a chicken *after* it has been cooked, so that the chicken won't be dry and hard. Or you may simply wrap skinned chicken in aluminum foil to prevent loss of juices during cooking.)

If you cook lean meat, fish, or poultry properly, you can eat generous portions without worrying about the calories or the fat. The hidden fat in lean meat won't do you any harm if you eliminate all the visible fat. Actually, you must have some fat in your diet for the best of health. You should go easy on pork, though, since it contains a considerable amount of invisible saturated fat.

Broiling Is Best

Whenever possible, it's usually best to roast, bake, or broil your meats on a rack so that fat dripping from the meat can be collected in a bottom pan for disposal. Tough meats can be stewed or braised if all the visible fat is cut away before cooking. A little vinegar, lemon juice, or tomato juice in the cooking water will have a tenderizing effect.

As far as your reducing diet is concerned, it makes little difference whether the meat you eat is rare or well done. If you want to make sure that there are no live parasites in your meats, however, you should cook them at least medium well. You should *never* eat pork that has a pink color.

Fish Is Ideal for Dieters

Since fish is a good low-fat source of protein, it should be included in a reducing diet as often as possible. Try broiling it on a greased rack. Sprinkle it lightly with skimmed milk or tomato juice before cooking. Fish may also be "poached" (simmered gently in water in a covered pan) or baked.

How to Broil Chicken and Fish

Remove the skin from chicken before baking or broiling. Cut the bird into halves through the breastbone. Break the joints and cut off the wing tips. Sprinkle with salt. Bake in an oven at 400 degrees Fahrenheit for 45 minutes to one hour. Turn once during cooking.

When you broil chicken on a rack, place the bird about five inches above the heat and turn it as it browns so that it will cook evenly. Cook for 35 to 45 minutes. You can, of course, baste chicken with your favorite barbecue sauce.

Fish can be basted with tomato juice or clam juice to prevent drying. When broiling fillets (no more than 1 ½ inches thick), place them in a preheated broiling pan that is close to the heating unit. It takes only about five minutes to cook most fish. When fish is done, the flesh will change from a clear transparent color to creamy white. Fish that is cooked too much will turn yellow and become tough. Properly cooked fish is easily flaked with a fork.

Keep Variety in Your Cooking

There are many ways to cook meat, fish, and poultry to add variety to your meals. Stewing fish with vegetables, for example, makes a tasty dieter's dish. You can find many good recipes in a good low-fat, low-calorie cook book. Always remember, however, that it's best to use *simple cooking methods* in preparing natural foods for good health and an ideal bodyweight.

A Special Note for Psoriasis Victims

If you suffer from psoriasis, it might be a good idea to *boil* your meats, fish, and poultry for ten minutes before roasting, baking, or broiling. This will eliminate taurine, a non-essential amino acid that may aggravate psoriasis. Remember, however, that boiling meats results in a loss of B vitamins. So if you must boil your meats, it might be a good idea to take a Vitamin B-complex supplement. This can be purchased in any drug store or health food store without a prescription.

When you boil meats in soup, always chill the soup and skim off the hard surface fat. Rewarm the soup just before serving.

Meat substitutes made from soybeans are rich in protein but low in taurine. If you must reduce your intake of meat because you have psoriasis or for some other reason, try to include soybean products in your diet.

Unsweetened gelatin is a good source of low-fat protein; but since it does not contain all the essential amino acids you cannot rely upon it as a sole source of protein. It can, however, be used along with other foods to help fill your stomach with low-calorie bulk and to help meet your protein requirements.

DON'T COOK WITH OILS

Many people feel that it's all right to fry foods in vegetable oil, since oil is an unsaturated fat. Frying in any type of oil, however, adds fattening calories. Furthermore, when vegetable oil is heated to temperatures above 215 degrees centigrade for 15 minutes or longer, the fatty acids begin to break down into a toxic cancer-causing substance. If you use a little cold-pressed vegetable oil on your green salads, as I suggested earlier, you'll get the essential fatty acids you need without using vegetable oil as cooking oil. It won't be necessary to use butter or margarine, either, except possibly in small amounts on your whole-grain breakfast toast. Remember, however, that the vegetable oil in margarine has been hardened by a process called hydrogenation. This means that *hard* margarines may be just as harmful to your arteries as saturated fat. The softer a margarine is, the higher the percentage of essential fatty acids or unsaturated fat.

If you must use a little margarine on your breakfast toast, and you don't like to use vegetable oil on your salads, you might want to mix vegetable oil (preferably safflower oil or corn oil) into margarine to increase its content of essential fatty acids. (Keep the mixture in a refrigerator so that it won't be too liquid to spread on toast.) There's nothing wrong with using a little butter occasionally, since it contains natural Vitamins A and D and helps satisfy your appetite. Just remember that too much oil or butter can add fattening calories. If you eliminate the high-calorie refined carbohydrates as I instructed you to do, you can stand a few calories from vegetable oil or butter.

EGGS SHOULD BE A PART OF YOUR DIET

Eggs can be an important part of your reducing diet if you aren't having trouble with your blood cholesterol. Some nutritionists maintain that the lecithin in egg yolk that has not been subjected to a high temperature can counteract the cholesterol in the yolk. If this is true, it would be best to soft boil your eggs so that there won't be enough heat to destroy the essential fatty acids in the yolk. Eggs are a good source of high-quality protein, and the yolks supply fat-soluble vitamins that tend to be deficient in a low-fat diet. If other sources of animal fat are reduced, I do not feel that an egg or two a day will have any harmful effects on your blood cholesterol. Besides, if your diet contains adequate amounts of B vitamins and essential fatty acids, your body should be able to control the amount of fat and cholesterol in your blood. Take your choice of scrambled, poached, or soft-boiled eggs.

Note: Do not eat raw eggs. Raw egg white contains avidin, a substance that prevents absorption of the B vitamin biotin. Raw eggs may also be diseased. Cooking an egg destroys avidin as well as any germs that might have penetrated a cracked shell. Properly cooked eggs are wholesome and healthful.

How to Prepare Eggs without Fat

The best and easiest way to prepare an egg is to boil it. First wash the egg. Then place it in a pot of cold water. Heat the water slowly to simmering. Cover the pot, remove it from the stove, and let it stand for three minutes. Plunge the egg into cold water before serving.

To poach an egg, bring a little salty water to a boil in a shallow pan. Break the egg into a saucer and then slip it into the water. Reheat the water to simmering and then cover the pan and remove it from the stove. Leave the egg in the water for about five minutes—or until the egg is firm.

HOW TO IMPROVE YOUR HEALTH AND REDUCE YOUR BODYWEIGHT WITH BREAD

Natural whole-grain cereals and breads supply Vitamin E, bran, and other essential elements that help you fight fat. There is now some evidence to indicate that the bran in whole-grain products may actually help you reduce. One researcher noted in a December, 1973, issue of *Lancet,* a British medical journal, that fiber in the diet actually reduced absorption of calories. Subjects on a high-fiber diet, for example, absorbed only 92.5 percent of food calories as compared to 97 percent in subjects on a low-residue diet. Volunteers who ate whole-grain breads excreted 321 calories a day through bowel action. Subjects who ate white bread excreted only 99 calories a day.

Other research indicates that extra roughage in the diet may also lower blood cholesterol, even when the diet is high in fat. In one study involving a group of men who ate a high-fat diet for 10 weeks and then ate the same diet supplemented with extra roughage for the next 55 weeks, the average cholesterol level dropped from 206.4 milligrams to 160 milligrams. The doctors theorized that increased roughage in the intestinal tract increases excretion of bile salts, which the body forms from cholesterol. So putting extra bran into your diet might help reduce your bodyweight and lower your blood cholesterol as well as improve your bowel function.

You can find natural whole-grain breads and cereals (that do not contain additives or preservatives) in most supermarkets and in all health food stores. If you want to make sure that your bread is completely natural, you can make your own. You can increase the fiber content of the bread by mixing a few tablespoons of pure bran into the bread dough. *Or you may substitute one-half cup of coarse bran for an equal amount of flour.* Remember, however, that any kind of bread is fairly high in carbohydrate. You probably should not eat more than one slice with each meal unless you find that you can do so and still lose weight. There's one thing for sure: you *must* have some whole-grain products in a fat-disintegrator diet. And if you add a little extra bran to homemade bread, you'll reduce a little faster.

How to Make Homemade Bread

Here's a basic recipe for *whole-wheat* bread that should be simple to follow:

Mix 3 cups of warm water with ½ cup of honey and 2 packages of baker's yeast. Allow this mixture to stand for 5 minutes or longer and then add 5 cups of unsifted stone-ground whole-wheat flour.

Beat this mixture by hand 100 times or more.

Then add 2 or 3 cups more of whole-wheat flour (or enough to make the dough stiff) and 1 scant tablespoonful of salt.

Knead the dough until it is smooth and elastic, adding enough flour to prevent sticking.

Place the dough in an oiled bowl, in a warm place, and let the dough rise until it doubles in bulk.

Knead the dough back to its original size and place it in two 1 ½-pound loaf pans that have been greased with margarine.

Let the dough rise until it reaches the top of the pan before placing it in the oven.

Bake in a preheated oven at 350 degrees for about 60 minutes or until the bread is well browned.

SPROUTS PROVIDE CONCENTRATED FAT-FIGHTING NUTRIENTS

If you consistently eat fresh, natural foods, you can be *healthier*, even though you eat less and take in fewer calories.

Sprouts are tremendously rich in vitamins, and they make a tasty addition to all types of dishes, especially soups and salads. So be sure to include them occasionally in your reducing diet.

How to Grow Vitamin-Rich Sprouts

Sprouts can be produced from a variety of seeds and beans. Alfalfa sprouts are tasty and easy to grow. Get some alfalfa seeds from your health food store and follow this procedure:

Put about two tablespoons of seeds into a half-gallon large-mouthed jar. Tie a piece of old stocking over the mouth of the jar. Rinse the seeds, drain the water, and then rotate the jar in a horizontal position so that the seeds will stick to the walls of the jar. This will allow proper ventilation. Let the jar rest on its side in a warm, dark place.

It's very important to rinse the seeds several times daily so that you wash away molds and bacteria.

The seeds should be fully sprouted in about three days. Further growth can be stopped by putting the jar of sprouts in a refrigerator. Sprouts that are allowed to grow too long may lose their delicate flavor.

Note: Potato sprouts are poisonous; don't eat them!

YOGURT IS DIET FOOD SUPREME

Yogurt made from skimmed milk is another highly nourishing low-fat food that has many healthful benefits in a reducing diet. One researcher, for example, found that yogurt can actually *lower* blood cholesterol, even when made from cholesterol-rich whole milk. In order to reduce calories, however, it's best to make your yogurt from skimmed milk.

In addition to supplying calcium and protein, yogurt supplies the intestinal tract with bacteria that improve digestion and elimination. Yogurt with fresh fruit makes a nearly complete meal. Have it as often as possible. Use the acidophilus variety whenever possible.

Buttermilk, kefir, and kumiss are fermented milk products that can be susbstituted for yogurt.

How to Make Low-Calorie Yogurt

To make your own yogurt, add a little acidophilus culture to skimmed milk and then leave the mixture in a warm place until it thickens, usually eight to twelve hours. You can speed the development of yogurt by placing small containers of milk and culture in a pan of water that's maintained at a temperature of up to 110 degrees Fahrenheit. An electric frying pan may be useful for this purpose. I have used a closed box containing an electric light bulb. If you purchase a commercial yogurt starter in a health food store, just follow the instructions on the package.

When the yogurt is custard-like, place it in a refrigerator. If it is left out too long, it will become watery. Remember, however, that the longer yogurt stays in the refrigerator the more acid it becomes. If you prefer a mild yogurt, don't make more than you can eat in a week's time.

Once you have a supply of yogurt on hand, you can make new yogurt by adding one tablespoonful of yogurt to a pint of milk. Eventually, however, you'll have to start over with a new or fresh culture.

If you haven't yet developed a taste for yogurt, try eating it with fresh fruit, sliced tomatoes, frozen orange juice, or chopped onions. It will make a fresh, stimulating snack that will satisfy your appetite as well as fight fat.

MENTAL AIDS IN DIETING

If you stick to natural foods that are properly prepared, chances are you won't have any trouble controlling your appetite. There are, however, a few psychological gimmicks you can use to trick your stomach into accepting *smaller portions*. If you have only one slice of whole-grain bread with each meal, for example, cut it in half so that you'll have *two* pieces of bread. Reaching for the second piece will help satisfy your habit of having "seconds."

Using a *small plate* will give you the illusion of eating more. Then, when you clean your plate, you'll finish your meal with the satisfaction of knowing that you did not waste any food or eat too much. Most people cannot leave food on a plate, even if it means stuffing in hundreds of extra calories.

Eating slowly will also help satisfy your appetite with less food. Chewing each bite of food at least 25 times will improve digestion, aid in the absorption of nutrients, and give your appetite mechanism plenty of time to register. Try using a *small spoon or fork* so that you won't be able to get much food into your mouth at one time.

Although I have said repeatedly that you can eat generous portions of natural foods, you should learn to satisfy your appetite with *less* food whenever possible. Many people overeat simply because of bad eating habits rather than because they crave food. You'll learn in Chapter 6 how to shrink your stomach with an occasional fast so that it won't take much food to provide you with the satisfaction of a full stomach.

How Martin P. Cut Down without Cutting Out

Martin P. lost 12 pounds the first month when he strictly limited his diet to natural foods. Weight loss slowed up after a couple of months, however, and by the end of the third month he was still 15 pounds over his ideal weight. "I'm eating nothing but natural foods," Martin complained, "but I can't seem to lose that last 15 pounds."

I explained to Martin that it was always harder to lose the last few pounds. And since he had already lost 16 pounds, he would have to decrease his calorie intake in order to lose more weight. Martin was eating all the proper foods in a properly prepared balanced diet, so I advised him to eat smaller portions of all the basic foods rather than cut out some of his fruits and vegetables. With a few simple tricks such as using a smaller plate, Martin once again started losing a pound or two a week. He lost 15 pounds during the next three months. He lost a total of 31 pounds in six months, reducing his bodyweight from 191 pounds to 160—an ideal weight for him.

"I feel much better since I've started eating less," Martin reported, "and I seem to be getting all I need to eat. In fact, I don't believe I crave food as much as I once did." Martin was obviously getting all the nutrients his body needed. And since his stomach was smaller than it used to be, he simply could not hold as much food.

If your weight loss seems to slow down after a few months of eating all you want of natural foods, cut down on the amount of food you eat. Remember, however, that you should still eat some of all the basic foods. Once all the excess fat is gone, it will never come back. Your bodyweight will normalize without you making any further changes in your diet.

SUMMARY

1. Properly prepared natural foods will retain the nutrients you need to stay healthy on a reducing diet.

2. Fruits should always be eaten raw, but some vegetables yield more nutrients when they are cooked.

3. Vegetables should be cooked with as little heat and water as possible for as short a cooking time as possible—preferably by steaming.

4. Natural foods should always be prepared in a simple manner, with nothing added but a small amount of salt and pepper.

5. It's best to *broil* meat, chicken, and fish so that fat can drip into a bottom pan for disposal.

6. You can use a small amount of cold-pressed vegetable oil on a green salad, but you should not use oils in cooking.

7. Raw salads and whole-grain bread prepared at home supply essential nutrients as well as fiber and bran that aid elimination and reduce absorption of calories.

8. Yogurt and sprouts are highly nourishing foods that can complement any reducing diet.

9. Eggs are best poached or soft boiled so that fat-fighting essential fatty acids won't be destroyed by excessive heat.

10. You can reduce a tendency to overeat by using a small plate and a small spoon and then chewing each bite of food at least 25 times.

5

How to Stay
on a Fat-Disintegrator Diet
When Dining Out

It's always best to eat at home whenever possible, so that you can prepare your own foods. This way, you can make sure that you get more nutrients and less calories. You can also do a better job of controlling your intake of sugar and fat in order to protect your arteries and prolong your life.

Few of us can avoid eating out occasionally, however, especially when we travel. And when we entertain guests and friends, it's sometimes necessary to "dine out" in order to "make the proper impression." Unfortunately, too many people *entertain* themselves by eating at all the "new places." Dining out becomes a form of recreation.

In many cases, the pleasure of eating is substituted for unfulfilled gratification in love, work, hobbies, and other personal activities. When you eat for reasons other than to satisfy your appetite and to nourish your body, you are simply taking calories that must be stored as body fat. So if you do dine out, do so only when you are hungry, not when you are bored, lonely, or disappointed. And don't get into the habit of eating out just to entertain yourself.

The Case of Faye and Eddie

Eddie and Faye J. were both suffering from chronic back trouble when I suggested that they each lose about 25 pounds. "Cut out refined and processed foods," I suggested, "and eat more lean meats and fresh vegetables. You'll have less back trouble if you'll lose a few pounds." A few months later, they were back in my office with a backache. Both of them had *gained* a couple of pounds. "I don't know why we haven't lost any weight," Faye complained. "We've been trying to eat natural foods."

I learned that Eddie and Faye rarely prepared their own meals. They both ate in cafeterias and restaurants just about every day. When I explained to them how restaurants often increase the calorie content of foods while destroying nutrients, they agreed to prepare their own meals as often as possible and then carefully select their foods when they dine out. It took Faye only two months to lose 25 pounds. It took Eddie a little longer to lose that much weight, since he could not resist an occasional beer.

"You were right, Doctor," Eddie reported. "We're having less back trouble since we lost some weight. And since we've started preparing more meals at home, we feel better and have more energy. We're getting plenty of exercise, too," he said with a wink, "since we're getting a lot more loving."

Most of what I told Eddie and Faye is outlined in this chapter. If you eat out often, study this chapter carefully, even if you don't have a backache. I won't guarantee that eating at home will help your love life, but it will certainly help solve your weight problem.

HOW COOKS KILL FOODS

When you eat food prepared by someone else, you can never be sure of what you're getting. Vegetables prepared in restaurants, for example, are often seasoned with sugar and fat in order to make them taste better. And if they have been boiled and left on a steam table for very long, they may not have much nutritional value. Prolonged exposure to heat, light, water, and air can literally reduce a vegetable to empty bulk that contains nothing but calories. Raw salads that have been shredded many hours before you eat them also lose many of their nutrients. Meats and vegetables that have been fried or cooked in oil are often left soaking in oil—until they become too greasy to eat. I never could understand why all cooks do not drain off excess grease from freshly fried foods. Simply laying fried chicken on a couple of paper towels, for example, would eliminate much harmful cooking fat.

COOKING-FATS CAN KILL YOU!

Everyone knows that too much fat in the diet clogs arteries and contributes to overweight. There are other dangers in fried foods. Heating cooking oil to a high temperature results in a breakdown of fatty acids, and a harmful, toxic substance is formed that can upset the stomach and contribute to the development of cancer. *Cooking oils should be used only once and then be discarded.* Yet, many restaurants use the same oil over and over. How many times have you ordered fried chicken that tasted like shrimp or fish?

When cooking oils are heated excessively, they begin to smoke. And when they are used repeatedly, they smoke at a lower temperature, which indicates that the fatty acids in the oil are deteriorating. Vegetable oils have a higher smoking temperature than animal fats. This is one reason why you should use vegetable oil when you find it necessary to cook with oil. Remember, however, that fried foods contribute extra calories. And when vegetable oil is heated, the fatty acids that combat hardening of the arteries are destroyed. So be sure to avoid fried foods as much as possible, even when they're fried in vegetable oil.

CHOOSE FOODS CAREFULLY

Many foods served in restaurants have been prepared in such a way that they *gain* calories and *lose* nutrients. A steady diet of such foods will result in an overweight but undernourished body. Without adequate nutrients, fat in the diet cannot be converted into energy. This is one reason why you'll *feel better* if you prepare *fresh* foods at home. When you do dine out, keep these basic foods in mind: raw salads, cottage cheese, lean meat, eggs, fish, poultry, vegetables, fresh fruits and melons, milk, and juices. *You should avoid breads and cereals, since they will usually be of the refined variety.* Breakfast should not be too much of a problem, since you can get ham, eggs, and oatmeal or grits in most restaurants. You can also order fruit or vegetable juice. Unfortunately, many short-order cooks use far too much grease in frying or scrambling eggs, which adds extra calories and harmful oil.

Remember that you must eliminate sugar, white flour, processed foods, and fried foods in order to lose weight without going on a low-calorie diet.

No Limit on Salads

When you eat buffet style in a cafeteria or restaurant, you can literally "load up" with raw salads, such as lettuce and tomatoes or carrots and celery. Avoid fruit salads that have been made with canned fruit. Try to include something raw at both noon and evening meals. Salads containing a small amount of avocado will supply the essential fatty acids you need to burn body fat.

Look for Low-Fat Meats

When you select a meat, look for something like roast beef, broiled fish, or baked chicken. Find something that's not fried or buried in gravy or grease. You can eat a generous portion of lean meat, chicken, or fish if it is not fat or greasy. If you must have fried chicken, peel off the grease-soaked skin and discard it.

Pick at Least One Vegetable

One vegetable will be enough to balance your meal if you have a raw salad. Just be sure to pick a vegetable that's not submerged in water or oil. A vegetable that has been prepared in a simple manner and has not been camouflaged in a fancy dish is best.

When you have selected meat, chicken, or fish and two vegetables, or one vegetable and a salad, you'll have all you need for a good meal. A broiled steak, a baked potato, and a tossed salad, for example, is a good bet when dining out.

Be Careful with Breads and Beverages

If you can't find a corn muffin that's not greasy, you can skip the bread. Very few restaurants serve pure whole-grain bread. And if you can't get milk or juice, you can drink water. If you're extremely overweight, or if you have a blood cholesterol problem, you may have to skip the milk if you can't get skimmed milk. I do not recommend tea or coffee, since they contain stimulants that may indirectly lower your blood sugar and speed the storage of blood sugar as fat. I do not recommend the use of artificial sweeteners, either, since they may be harmful to your health. You can do without artificial sweeteners, just as you can do without sugar.

Look for Natural Desserts

You can skip desserts when you dine out—unless you can find raw fruit, sliced melon, cantaloupe, or sliced Cheddar cheese. Whenever possible, it's always a good idea to finish a meal with a piece of raw fruit, especially when traveling, since chewing fruit helps clean your teeth. I frequently grab a handful of carrot sticks or celery stalks to chew on after a meal for the sole purpose of cleaning my teeth.

If you *must* have something sweet after a meal, eat a little dried fruit after you leave the restaurant. You can purchase pocket-size boxes of raisins in any grocery store, or you may simply carry a box in your coat pocket. Fruit sugar is more complex and less fattening then refined sugar, and there is some evidence to indicate that fruit sugar (fructose) will not trigger a pancreatic reaction the way refined sugar does. But since dried fruits are rich in calories, you shouldn't eat them except in small amounts following a regular meal.

Choosing Between Fresh and Frozen Foods

Whenever you buy your own vegetables, you should always select *fresh* vegetables, since they are likely to contain more nutrients. Frozen vegetables can be very nourishing, but the handling and preparation of such vegetables from the time they are harvested until they reach your plate, especially in a restaurant, can result in the loss of many essential nutrients. Even if a vegetable is properly frozen, time alone will result in the destruction of sensitive vitamins. Frozen beans, broccoli, cauliflower, and spinach, for example, lose one-third to three-fourths of their Vitamin C in a year. Once frozen vegetables are allowed to thaw and are then refrozen, as often happens in the handling and storage of such vegetables, there may be very little left but calories and bulk. And after frozen vegetables are boiled, overheated, and left exposed to heat, light, and air on a steam table, they may be of no value to you in keeping you lean and healthy. So if you do have to eat in restaurants frequently, it might be a good idea to take a good vitamin and mineral supplement. Remember that *good health* is essential in maintaining the metabolic balance your body needs to help *prevent* an abnormal build-up of body fat. Some unhealthy persons, for example, tend to build-up excess body fat on low-calorie diets that would keep the average person lean. And when there is a deficiency in water-soluble B vitamins and other nutrients, the body cannot easily "burn off" stored fat. These are only a few of the reasons why it's so important to eat fresh, properly prepared foods.

Note: If you purchase frozen vegetables for use at home, be sure to select those that do not show evidence of thawing. Then cook them as soon as possible. It's always best to drop a frozen vegetable into boiling water to prevent loss of nutrients from slow thawing. Of course, boiling a vegetable may result in the loss of water-soluble vitamins if you do not use the cooking water as soup. Steaming a vegetable, as suggested in Chapter 4, will eliminate many of the destructive effects of cooking.

Even canned vegetables lose nutrients when they rest on warm shelves for many months. And they are just as sensitive to improper cooking and handling as any other type of vegetable. Actually, it matters very little whether a vegetable is fresh, frozen, or canned if it is not properly prepared. The end result is the same: bulk containing only empty calories. Very few restaurants serve fresh vegetables, and the vegetables are almost always improperly prepared.

FOODS LOSE NUTRIENTS IN MANY WAYS

Properly prepared fresh vegetables should retain most of their natural color, but watch out for the brightly colored vegetables served in some fancy restaurants. Many professional cooks add acids or alkalis to vegetables in order to preserve their color. Adding a little baking soda to the cooking water of green vegetables, for example, preserves their color but destroys Vitamin C and makes the vegetables mushy. Red vegetables retain their color better when vinegar or lemon juice is added to the cooking water, but this procedure hardens the vegetables and increases cooking time. You already know that the longer you cook a vegetable the more vitamins it loses.

There are many "gourmet" cooking methods that result in pretty dishes, and most of them decrease the nutritional value of vegetables. The practice of boiling rice and other vegetables and then pouring off the water and rinsing them for better separation, for example, is a bad practice that results in the loss of many vitamins. Some restaurants pour hot water over leftover vegetables to warm them, washing away more of the water-soluble vitamins.

Even milk loses nutrients when left exposed to light. Milk exposed to sunlight loses more than 40 percent of its riboflavin (one of the B vitamins) in a couple of hours. If the temperature of the milk rises above 70 degrees Fahrenheit, the loss increases. Keep your milk cold in a dark refrigerator. Paper containers or brown glass will help protect against the effects of light.

Dehydrated eggs lose nutrients more readily than fresh eggs. When stored at room temperature, for example, they lose two-thirds of their Vitamin A in nine months. This may be the case in the use of many other powdered or dehydrated foods served in restaurants.

There are obviously many good reasons why you should prepare *fresh* foods at home, using simple cooking methods, rather than eat out. When you eat food prepared by someone else, you have no assurance that you're getting the nutrients you need to combat the craving that leads to overeating and over-weight. When you prepare your own foods at home, you can at least make sure that what you eat is fresh and wholesome.

A POINT WORTH REPEATING

Remember that on a reducing diet in which you must eat smaller portions, it's absolutely essential that you eat foods that are rich in vitamins and minerals. You cannot afford to depend upon poorly cooked or leftover foods that supply little more than empty calories.

"FAST" ON RAW FOODS WHEN YOU TRAVEL

Traveling affords a good opportunity to "clean out" your system by eating fresh fruit, cheese, nuts, seeds, raw vegetables, whole-grain products, and other natural, uncooked foods. It also provides a good opportunity for a small amount of fasting. When you eat less for a couple of days, your stomach shrinks, reducing your appetite for larger amounts of foods. You'll learn more about fasting in Chapter 6.

I usually do not recommend total fasting—never more than two days at a time. When you do "fast," it may be a good idea to eat fruits and drink juices and other liquids. The acid in fruits will alkalize your urine and help combat a build-up of harmful acids in your system.

Note: Although most fruits contain acid, they have an alkaline reaction in your system. When they are digested and metabolized, they leave an alkaline ash. Plums, prunes, cranberries, and raw rhubarb are the only fruits I know of that have an *acid* reaction in your system, adding acid to your urine. Meat, bread, potatoes, eggs, cereals, and foods of that type contribute acid to your system. When you fast longer than 48 hours, burning of body fat releases acid into your system. This is why I recommend the use of fruits and juices on a "fasting diet."

Try a Two-Day Fruit Diet

The next time you take a trip, and you want to avoid eating questionable foods prepared in restaurants and cafeterias, take advantage of the situation and go on a "fruit diet" to cleanse your system. It'll fit right in with your reducing diet, and chances are you'll eat *less* when you resume your normal diet.

Eat a variety of fruits along with a little cottage cheese or yogurt. Raw vegetables such as carrots, tomatoes, celery, lettuce, and cabbage will help balance your snacks. A few seeds or nuts will supply essential fatty acids along with protein. Any health food store can supply you with pumpkin seeds, sunflower seeds, cashew nuts, almonds, and other raw seeds and nuts. Just about every grocery store stocks raw peanuts.

Fruit and vegetable juices can be found in the coolers of convenience food stores all along the highway. Skim milk can often be found in pint containers. Remember that vegetable juice has fewer calories than milk or fruit juice. You can make up a fairly good diet with cheese, nuts, seeds, juices, milk, and raw fruits and vegetables. Or you may simply eat fresh fruits for a couple of days.

Although fruits, seeds, and nuts are fairly high in calories, it's not likely that you'll get an excessive number of calories from these natural foods if you do not eat cooked foods. Your appetite mechanism will tell you when you have had enough. Just eat when you feel hungry. *Stop* eating when you feel satisfied.

The Story About the Traveling Salesman

Carlos T. had been a traveling salesman for only two years. During that time, his weight increased from a lean 160 to a fat

210. "I don't know why I'm gaining so much weight," he said with obvious dismay. "I don't eat nearly as much as I did when I ate at home."

It was easy to see why Carlos was gaining weight. In addition to being less active, he was eating more snacks, sandwiches, and other refined foods that were high in calories and low in nutrients. Although he was eating less, he was taking in more calories and burning fewer calories. I told Carlos how to select certain basic foods in restaurants and cafeterias and then suggested that he occasionally alternate cooked meals with snacks of raw foods. I told him all the things I have already told you in this chapter. When he came in for his checkup at the end of the month, he had lost about 10 pounds. "I actually ate more this month than I did last month," he beamed, "and I still lost 10 pounds. Even my friends have noticed that I'm looking slimmer. I certainly feel better. And I don't feel so sluggish and bloated."

"Keep eating wholesome, natural foods as I instructed you to do and you'll lose *all* of your excess fat," I advised Carlos. "You'll discover new pleasures in eating, and you'll experience a great improvement in health."

If you were in my office, I would tell you the same thing.

A Final Caution for Traveling Fasters

You probably should not stay on a "fasting" or raw food diet for more than a few days. You need cooked meat, eggs, and other animal products for iron, protein, Vitamin B_{12}, and other essential nutrients. Also, some vegetables yield more nutrients when they are properly cooked than when they are raw.

If you must travel in your job, try to eat at places where they serve wholesome "home-cooked" meals—where fresh *natural* foods are prepared.

CARRY A LUNCH TO WORK

Persons who must punch a clock for a living and are unable to eat noon meals at home might prefer to carry a lunch rather than eat in a restaurant. A simple meat or egg sandwich on pure whole-wheat bread, along with a raw carrot or a couple of celery sticks and a piece of fresh fruit, will provide a nutritious, low-calorie meal. Fresh fruit during a rest break can be refreshing as well as delicious, and it will give your blood sugar an energizing boost.

There are endless combinations of natural foods that can be used in preparing low-calorie lunch-box meals. Boiled eggs, baked chicken, cottage cheese and fresh fruit, and whole raw vegetables such as tomatoes, carrots, and celery are popular lunch-box items. If skimmed milk or juices aren't available, plain water can be used as a beverage with your meal. If you are really hungry, you'll find that simple, natural foods will "hit the spot." And if you are really thirsty, a glass of cool water will be more satisfying than a bottled beverage.

The important thing to remember is not to include any refined or processed foods in your lunch box. Lunch meats on white bread, for example, are a no-no. Canned fruits often contain sugar, and they are not as nourishing as fresh fruit.

Pack your lunch box with completely natural foods and rediscover the *real* taste of food. You'll be rewarded with better health as well as a leaner body.

Remember that *overeating* can have harmful effects on both your mind and your body. You can think better and work better if your stomach is not completely full. So don't make the mistake of packing your lunch box—and your stomach—until it is too full.

SUMMARY

1. Food prepared in restaurants is often deficient in nutrients but rich in calories, making it difficult to control your bodyweight when you dine out.

2. When you do dine out, always select simple, natural foods—such as broiled chicken, baked potato, and salad—that are not swimming in grease or water.

3. If you can't find such simple desserts as raw fruit, melon, or cantaloupe, skip the dessert—or take along a pocket-size box of dried fruit.

4. Whenever possible, dine where it is a policy to use *fresh* vegetables rather than frozen or canned vegetables.

5. Avoid fancy dishes that have bright colors or unknown ingredients.

6. Don't be afraid to ask a restaurant waitress if foods such as milk, eggs, and mashed potatoes are fresh rather than powdered.

7. When you travel, it's often a good idea to "fast" on a diet of fresh fruit, cheese, raw vegetables, and other uncooked foods for a day or two.

8. Cottage cheese and fresh fruit, along with a raw vegetable and a handful of seeds or nuts, will provide a fairly well-balanced meal.

9. It's never a good idea to fast or go on an unbalanced restaurant diet for more than a couple of days at a time.

10. In many cases, it may be best for "working folks" to pack a lunch box for the noon meal and then prepare a balanced evening meal at home.

6

How to Keep Slim
with Special Fat Controllers

When you have succeeded in reducing your bodyweight, there are a few simple measures that you can employ to avoid regaining the lost weight. An occasional short fast, for example, will help curb your appetite by shrinking your stomach. Keeping a record of everything you eat will help you determine how many calories and how much carbohydrate you are taking in. Double-checking your diet for possible causes of hypoglycemia or low blood sugar will assure you better control over your body's energy-burning, fat-storing mechanism. All of these measures have been discussed briefly in previous chapters of this book. In this chapter, you'll get all the details of how to go on a fast, how to measure the amount of carbohydrate in your diet, and how to make sure that you don't ever suffer from the fattening fatigue of hypoglycemia. If you can learn to use these fat-controlling measures effectively, you'll have a better chance of staying slim for the rest of your life.

HOW TO FAST EFFECTIVELY

When most people think of fasting, they think of a long period of starvation. Actually, fasting for an improvement in health simply means *reducing* your food intake for a short period of time. It's not necessary or desirable to quit eating completely. Nor is it necessary to fast for a long period of time. If you're used to eating large meals, you may have to begin reducing the amount of food you eat each day for several days in order to shrink your stomach a little before you actually begin fasting. A sudden and drastic reduction in the amount of food you eat may result in hunger pangs caused by contractions of an empty stomach. Production of stomach acid triggered by hunger might inflame your stomach or produce intestinal discomfort.

Gradually reduce the size of your meals for a week. Then, for two days, eat nothing but fresh fruits and raw vegetables. You can drink all the fruit and vegetable juice you want. Plenty of liquids will help flush out wastes. Remember that vegetable juice has fewer calories than fruit juice.

It's better to eat and drink small amounts frequently throughout the day rather than eat only at mealtime. Eat when you feel hungry. You'll be surprised at how little you need to satisfy your appetite when you eat raw fruits and vegetables.

Note: If you suffer from diabetes, stomach ulcers, or some other illness, check with your doctor before making any drastic changes in your diet.

Why You Need Fruits and Vegetables on a "Fasting Diet"

There are good reasons for eating raw fruits and vegetables when you "fast." If you go on a total fast and eat nothing or drink nothing but water, hunger may be agonizing. And if a total fast is continued for longer than two days, depletion of glycogen stores will force the body to depend entirely upon stored fat for energy. When this happens, hunger disappears. Excessive burning of body fat, however, may overload the blood and the kidneys with acid waste products, resulting in gout and other forms of illness. A person living totally off body fat and tissue protein can literally starve himself to death without suffering from hunger. Of course, no one would fast for such a long period of time. But any fast lasting for more than a couple of days may result in nutritional deficiencies that could damage your health.

Even when you eat fruits and vegetables, it's best not to "fast" longer than two days.

Raw fruits and vegetables supply cellulose that will quiet hunger pains and sweep away wastes and residues that have accumulated in your intestinal tract. They will also combat a build-up of acid in your system. *Chewing* raw foods will help prevent absorption of bone around the roots of your teeth. Persons who go on prolonged "juice diets" may develop periodontal disease from lack of exercise for their teeth and gums. No bulk or fiber in the bowels may also result in constipation.

After a short fast, when you begin to resume eating meats, cereals, and other basic foods that should be part of a balanced diet, it won't take much food to satisfy your appetite. Your stomach will have shrunken so much that it simply cannot hold much food. Of course, as the months go by, you'll probably stretch your stomach again by eating progressively larger amounts of food. When you begin to notice that you're overeating and gaining weight, you can again taper your food intake down to a two-day fast. As long as the fast does not last for more than two days, you need not worry about developing a nutritional deficiency, especially if you satisfy your appetite with fresh fruits and raw vegetables.

How Cindy Used a Fast to Reduce Her Bodyweight

Cindy K. had been on a natural foods fat-disintegrator diet for several months. She had been losing about five pounds a month and had already lost 25 pounds. She enjoyed eating, however, and she felt that it took far too much food to satisfy her appetite. When she stepped on the scales and found that she had lost only two pounds in a month, she knew she was eating too much. I advised her to try the fasting procedure described in this chapter. "A two-day fast once a month," I suggested, "will shrink your stomach so that you won't have to eat so much to satisfy your appetite."

When Cindy completed her fast and resumed a balanced fat-disintegrator diet, she once again began to lose more than one pound a week. "Just a few more months," she beamed, "and I'll be down to my best weight. I felt so good during the fast, however, that I plan to fast once a month from now on."

HOW TO CONTROL YOUR CARBOHYDRATE INTAKE

Some reducing experts recommend that in order to lose weight you must take in no more than 1,600 calories with less than 75 grams of carbohydrate. You know from reading other chapters of this book that most people can lose weight simply by eating natural foods and eliminating refined and processed foods. If your pancreas has been sensitized by eating excessive amounts of sugar and refined carbohydrates, however, it may be necessary to reduce your intake of natural high-carbohydrate foods until that sensitivity disappears. Then, when your weight has been reduced, you can begin eating a little more carbohydrate.

If you keep a daily record of what you eat, you can get some idea of the number of calories you're taking in and the amount of carbohydrate your meals contain by checking with the calorie-carbohydrate tables in this chapter. You can never be sure of the exact calorie or carbohydrate value of any food, however, since it's difficult or impossible to measure foods exactly. So while you might make an effort to keep your carbohydrate intake down around 75 grams, it probably does not matter if you go over this figure a few grams if you eat strictly natural foods.

How a Professional Model Slimmed Down

If you eat properly prepared natural foods, it's very likely that your weight will normalize without you measuring the foods you eat. Losing a few extra pounds for that slim look, however, may be more difficult, making it necessary to begin paying attention to the calorie and carbohydrate content of your foods. Doris G., for example, was a professional model who wanted to lose a few extra pounds. She looked great to me, but she insisted that she was 10 pounds too heavy. I gave Doris a copy of a table listing the calorie and carbohydrate content of the basic natural foods and suggested that she try to avoid getting more than 75 grams of carbohydrate a day. Since she weighed 120 pounds and wanted to reduce to 110 pounds, I advised her to keep her calorie intake down around 1,300 calories. (Remember that to maintain a certain bodyweight, a fairly active woman needs at least 12 calories per pound of weight. To maintain a weight of 110 pounds, Doris needed 1,320 calories a day: 110 x 12 = 1,320.)

Doris lost the 10 pounds in about six weeks with no trouble at all.

TABLE GIVING THE CALORIE AND CARBO-HYDRATE CONTENT OF THE BASIC NATURAL FOODS

Basic Food Group	Measure	Number of Calories	Grams of Carbo-hydrate
Milk, skim	2 cups	176	26
Egg	1 medium	81	0
Meat, fish, fowl, lean	4 ounces	376	0
Vegetables:			
Deep green or yellow	2 servings	54	12
Other vegetables.........	2 servings	90	20
Fruits:			
Citrus	1 serving	43	10
Other fruits.............	2 servings	146	38
Bread, whole grain	2 slices	124	24
Butter or margarine	1 tablespoon	100	0
Total calories and carbohydrate		1,190	130

If you stick to the simple, basic foods listed in this table, you can use this as a general guide in figuring the *approximate* number of calories and grams of carbohydrate in your diet. If you want to figure your diet more closely, you can use the table listing a variety of commonly used natural foods.

TABLE OF CALORIES AND CARBOHYDRATE IN A VARIETY OF COMMONLY USED NATURAL FOODS*

Natural Food	Measure	Number of Calories	Grams of Carbo-hydrate
Apple, raw	1 medium	54	14
Apple juice	½ cup	47	12
Apple sause, unsweetened	½ cup	41	11
Asparagus, fresh	6-7 spears	20	4
Avocado	½ peeled	167	6
Bacon	12 strips	611	3
	2 strips	100	1
Bacon, Canadian	3 ½ ounces	277	trace
Banana	1 small	85	22
Barley	½ cup	349	79
Beans:			
Lima, fresh ....., ...	⅔ cup	111	20
Green snap, fresh	¾ cup	25	5
Bean sprouts, mung, raw	1 cup	35	7
Beef:			
Lean, pot-roasted	3 ½ ounces	170	0
Hamburger, lean, broiled	1 patty	109	0
Roast, lean round	2.8 ounces	145	0
Steak, lean round	2.9 ounces	152	0
Beets, cooked, drained	½ cup	32	7
Beet greens, cooked	⅔ cup	18	3
Bouillon cube	1 cube	2	trace
Bran	1 ounce	95	21
Brazil nuts, shelled	⅔ cup	654	11

* The average serving of meat, cut by the butcher, is 3 1/2 ounces. When the fat has been cut away for cooking, however, the serving will usually be less than 3 ounces. This is why servings of "lean meat," as listed on this chart, are often less than 3 ounces.

Natural Food	Measure	Number of Calories	Grams of Carbo-hydrate
Bread:			
Rye, American	1 slice	56	12
Whole wheat	1 slice	56	11
Broccoli, cooked	⅔ cup	26	5
Brussels sprouts	¾ cup	36	6
Butter	1 tablespoon	100	trace
Buttermilk (skim milk)	½ cup	36	5
Cabbage:			
Raw	3 x 5 in. wedge	24	5
Cooked	1 ⅔ cup	20	4
Cantaloupe	⅙ melon	30	8
Carrots:			
Raw	2 carrots	42	10
Cooked	⅔ cup	31	7
Cashew nuts, roasted	1 ounce	168	9
Cauliflower:			
Raw	1 cup	27	5
Cooked	1 cup	22	4
Celery:			
Raw	2 stalks	17	4
Cooked	¾ cup diced	14	3
Chard	⅔ cup	18	3
Cheese:			
Cheddar, unprocessed	3 ½ ounces	398	2
	1 ounce	120	1
Cottage, skim milk	3 ½ ounces	106	3
	1 ounce	30	1
Chicken:			
Light meat, no skin	3 ½ ounces	166	0
Dark meat, no skin	3 ½ ounces	176	0
Chickpeas, dry	½ cup	360	61
Coconut, fresh	1 cup shredded	346	9

Natural Food	Measure	Number of Calories	Grams of Carbohydrate
Collards, cooked	½ cup	33	5
Corn, on cob	1 small ear	91	21
Corn bread	2 muffins	215	35
Corn grits	½ cup	51	11
Cowpeas, cooked . . . . ·	⅔ cup	108	18
Crabs, steamed	3 ½ ounces	93	1
Cucumbers, raw, peeled	⅓ cucumber	14	3
Dandelion greens:			
Raw	1 cup	45	9
Cooked	½ cup	33	6
Dates, dried	½ cup pitted	274	73
Eggplant, boiled	3 ½ ounces	19	4
Eggs, raw or cooked	1 medium	81	trace
Endive or escarole, raw	3 ½ ounces	20	4
Fats, vegetable oil	1 tablespoon	110	0
Figs, raw	3 small	80	20
Hazelnuts	100 grams	634	17
Fish:			
Bluefish, broiled	3 ½ ounces	159	0
Cod, broiled	3 ½ ounces	170	0
Flounder, baked	3 ½ ounces	202	0
Halibut, broiled	3 ½ ounces	171	0
Mackerel, Atlantic, broiled . . .	3 ½ ounces	236	0
Salmon, broiled	3 ½ ounces	182	0
Swordfish, broiled	3 ½ ounces	174	0
Tuna fish, canned in water . . .	3 ½ ounces	127	0
Grapefruit	½ small	41	11
Grapefruit juice, no sugar	½ cup	41	10
Grapes, raw	⅔ cup	69	16
Grape juice, bottled	3 ½ ounces	66	17
Guavas, raw	1 large	62	15

Natural Food	Measure	Number of Calories	Grams of Carbo- hydrate
Honey	1 tablespoon	64	17
Honeydew melon, raw	1 ½ x 7 in. wedge	33	8
Kale, fresh, cooked	1 cup	39	6
Kohlrabi, cooked	⅔ cup	24	7
Lamb:			
Chop, lean, broiled	2.4 ounces	125	0
Leg, lean, roasted	3 ounces	121	0
Shoulder, lean, roasted	2.7 ounces	150	0
Lentils, cooked	3 ½ ounces	106	19
Lettuce	¼ head	13	3
Liver:			
Beef, raw	3 ½ ounces	140	5
Beef, fried	3 ½ ounces	229	5
Calf, fried	3 ½ ounces	261	4
Pork, fried	3 ½ ounces	241	3
Lobster, cooked	3 ½ ounces	95	trace
Mangos, raw	½ medium	66	17
Margarine, fortified	1 tablespoon	101	trace
Milk, cow:			
Whole	1 cup	160	12
Skimmed	1 cup	88	13
Mustard greens, cooked	⅔ cup	23	4
Nectarines, raw	1 small	64	17
Oatmeal, cooked	⅔ cup	55	10
Oils, salad or cooking	1 tablespoon	124	0
Okra, cooked	9 pods	29	6
Olives, pickled:			
Green	16 olives	116	1
Ripe, Mission	2 olives	37	trace
Onions:			
Raw	1 onion	38	9

Natural Food	Measure	Number of Calories	Grams of Carbo- hydrate
Cooked	½ cup	29	7
Oranges..................	1 small	49	12
Orange juice:			
Fresh	½ cup	45	11
Canned, no sugar	½ cup	48	11
Oysters, raw	5-8 medium	66	3
Papayas, raw..............	½ cup cubes	39	10
Parsley, raw	1 tablespoon	1	trace
Parsnips, cooked	⅔ cup	66	15
Peaches, raw..............	1 peach	38	10
Peanuts, roasted	⅔ cup	585	19
Peanut butter	1 tablespoon	87	3
Pears, raw	1 medium pear	61	15
Peas, green, cooked	⅔ cup	72	12
Pecans, shelled	1 cup halves	687	15
Peppers, green, raw	1 large	22	5
Pickles:			
Dill, cucumber	1 large	11	2
Sweet, cucumber	½ cup	146	37
Pineapple:			
Raw	¾ cup diced	52	14
Canned in juice	1 slice	58	15
Pineapple juice, no sugar.....	½ cup	55	14
Plums, raw	2 medium	48	12
Popcorn, popped	1 cup	54	10
Pork, fresh:			
Chop, lean................	2.6 ounces	195	0
Roast, lean	2.9 ounces	182	0
Picnic, lean	2.6 ounces	157	0
Pork, smoked ham:			
Ham, cooked, lean	3 ounces	157	0

Natural Food	Measure	Number of Calories	Grams of Carbo- hydrate
Ham, canned	3 ½ ounces	193	1
Potatoes:			
Baked in skin	1 medium	93	21
Boiled, peeled	1 medium	65	15
Prunes:			
Dried	⅔ cup	255	67
Cooked, no sugar	6 prunes	119	31
Prune juice, canned	½ cup	77	19
Radishes, raw	4 small	7	1
Raisins, seedless	1 tablespoon	29	8
Rhubarb, raw	¾ cup diced	16	4
Rice, brown, cooked	⅔ cup	119	26
Rutabagas, boiled	⅔ cup diced	35	8
Sauerkraut, canned	⅔ cup	18	4
Sausage, pork, cooked	3 ½ ounces	476	0
Scallops, steamed	3 ½ ounces	112	—
Shrimp, fried	3 ½ ounces	225	10
Soybeans, boiled	3 ½ ounces	103	7
Soybean flour, defatted	1 cup	326	38
Soybean products:			
Soybean milk	½ cup	33	2
Soybean curd	3 ½ ounces	72	2
Soybean sprouts, cooked	1 cup	38	4
Spinach:			
Raw	3 ½ ounces	26	4
Cooked	½ cup	23	4
Squash:			
Summer, cooked	½ cup diced	15	3
Winter, baked	3 ½ ounces	63	15
Strawberries, raw	⅔ cup	37	8

Natural Food	Measure	Number of Calories	Grams of Carbo-hydrate
Sweet potatoes:			
Baked in skin	1 small	141	33
Boiled in skin	½ medium	114	26
Tangerines	1 medium	46	11
Tomatoes:			
Raw	1 small	22	5
Canned or cooked	½ cup	23	5
Tomato juice, canned	½ cup	19	4
Turkey, roasted flesh	3 ½ ounces	190	0
Turnips:			
Raw	¾ cup diced	30	7
Cooked	⅔ cup diced	23	5
Turnip greens, boiled	⅔ cup	20	4
Veal cutlet, broiled	3 ½ ounces	234	0
Walnuts, chopped	1 tablespoon	52	1
Watermelon	3 ½ ounces	26	6
Wheat flour, whole	1 cup	333	71
Wheat germ	1 cup	363	47
Wild rice, raw	⅔ cup	353	75
Yeast, dried brewer's	1 tablespoon	22	3
Yogurt, partially skimmed . . .	⅓ cup	50	5

This table is only a partial list of natural foods—just to give you some idea of the calorie and carbohydrate content of the foods you eat. You can find a more comprehensive list of foods in *Nutrition in Health and Disease,* published by J.B. Lippincott of Philadelphia, or in the U.S. Department of Agriculture's *Composition of Foods,* Handbook No. 8. You may find that there is considerable variation in the different food tables, so about the most you can hope for is a rough estimate of the amount of carbohydrate your meals contain.

A Sample Menu Giving Calorie and Carbohydrate Values

Here is a sample low-calorie, low-carbohydrate menu of the type I recommend for my patients. Remember that you can eat the foods you like best if you select foods from all the basic food groups.

Breakfast	Calories	Grams of Carbohydrate
2 medium eggs, poached 163		1
3 ounces lean ham 157		0
1 slice whole-wheat bread 56		11
1 cup tomato juice 38		8
1 cup Sanka 0		0
Midmorning Snack		
½ small grapefruit 41		11
Lunch		
3½ ounces tuna packed in water . . . 127		0
¼ head of lettuce, 1 small tomato . . 35		8
1 slice whole-wheat bread 56		11
Water or unsweetened tea 0		0
Midafternoon Snack		
½ cup yogurt, from skimmed milk. 36		5
Dinner		
3 ounces of lean roast beef 165		0
¾ cup green snap beans 25		5
1 ⅔ cup cabbage 20		4
1 cup skimmed milk 88		13
Evening Snack		
½ medium apple 27		7
3 ounces cottage cheese 90		3

Total number of calories: 1,124
Total grams of carbohydrate: 87

Denise Austin

UltraArm Workout Plan

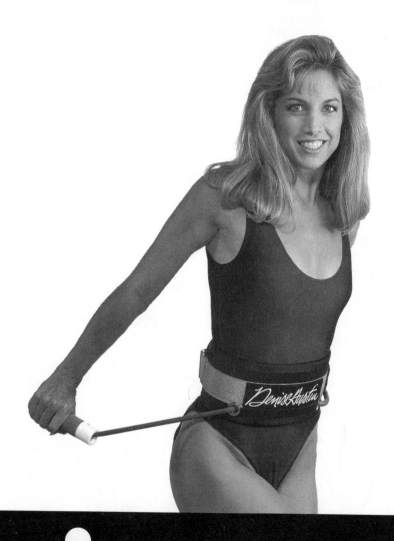

Bollinger

itness products for every body

Congratulations on investing in your UltraArm, the ultimate under arm firmer. I've designed this product to target tone the under arm muscle-the tricep. This muscle is the most under used muscle in the body and as a result it becomes soft and sometimes unattractive.

Just follow this program and you'll be be on your way to those beautiful arms you've always wanted.

Remember, I'm on ESPN every weekend morning with my show "Getting Fit With Denise Austin." Tune in and let's get fit together. You'll be so glad you did! And yes--you can do it!

Best always,

Denise Austin

Denise Austin

Stretching first is always best! Let's begin with the tricep stretch. Place your right hand in the middle of your shoulders behind your head. "Give yourself a pat on the back." Place your left hand on the right elbow. Push your right arm slowly down your back until you reach a point of tension. Feel a good stretch in your arm. (Never stretch to a point of pain.) Do not arch your back. Hold the stretch for 15 seconds. Relax and repeat with the other arm. *Benefit: Stretches the tricep.*

Upper Back Stretch

Put your right hand towards your left shoulde., Cup your right elbow with the palm of your left hand. Pull the elbow gently toward your left shoulder. Hold the stretch for 15 seconds. Then release. Switch sides. *Benefits: Stretches the upper back and releases tension.*

Do you ever feel tight in your shoulders? Muscle fibers "adapt" physiologically to states of increased tension. In other words, a muscle will eventually stay in a state of unhealthy tension unless you do something about it. To increase blood circulation and to ease tensed muscles, do what I do.

UltraArm Workout

Put your right hand on your left shoulder. Cup your right elbow with the palm of your left hand. Pull the elbow gently toward your left shoulder. Hold the stretch for 15 seconds, then release. Switch sides and pull your left elbow toward your right shoulder. Repeat. The benefit to you is this stretches and relaxes the muscles between your shoulder blades.

UltraArm Workout Plan.

Most of us don't work our triceps very much in normal daily activity. So the back of your upper arms tend to get flabby, but the triceps are important, both for appearances sake and for your overall level of strength.

Throughout my entire workout remember. "Do the best that you can do!" Good posture and technique is very important while using the UltraArm. Here are a few tips:
- -Always keep your knees slightly bent
- -Keep abdominal muscles tight
- -Exhale on the exertion (mostly when you extend the arm)
- -Just give it a "good try"

Level I-*Designed for the 1st 5 weeks. Beginner and way to maintain muscle tone.*

Level II-*Designed for the next 5 weeks or more. You may want to stay at this level.*

Level III-*For the challenged athlete.*

Denise Austin's UltraArm Workout can be done in 5 minutes. To see results do the workout at least 5 days a week.

Right Under-Arm Firmer

Hold the right handle with our right hand. Lift right elbow behind you and keep it stationary. Extend your arm pulling with resistance backwards. Then release slowly bending your elbow. *Benefit: Firms and strengthen the tricep muscles of the right arm.*

Level I- Do 5 Times.
Level II- Do 10 Times
Level III- Do 15 Times

Left Under-Arm Firmer

Hold the right handle with our left hand. Lift left elbow behind you and keep it stationary. Extend your arm pulling with resistance backwards, Then release slowly bending your elbow. Benefit: Firms and strengthen the tricep muscles of the left arm.

Level I- Do 5 Times.
Level II- Do 10 Times
Level III-Do 15 Times

Two-Arm Triceps Toner

Holding both handles, lift elbows up and back. Now pull with resistance to extend your arms. Release slowly. *Benefits: tones the tricep and posterior deltoid muscles. (Back of Shoulders)*

Level I- Do 5 Times.
Level II- Do 10 Times
Level III-Do 15 Times

Under-Arm Lift.

This exercise can be done with both arms of one at a time. Hold the handle with palms facing upward behind you 9 Palm of hand towards the ceiling). With arm/arms extended lift up an inch and down an inch- "pulsing" the movement up and down.

Try to keep arm/arms straight but not locked; elbows with a slight bend. *Benefits: Strengthens triceps posterior deltoids and upper back muscles.*

Level I- Do 5 Lifts.
Level II- Do 10 Lifts.
Level III-Do 15 Lifts.

That's it! The program that can tone and firm your under arms.
Let me know how it works for you!
Send comments and pictures to:

Denise Austin Marketing ,
222 W Airport Freeway, Irving TX 75062

Calories Do Count—and Carbohydrates, Too!

Some reducing experts maintain that it does not matter how many calories you take in if you limit your carbohydrate intake to less than 75 grams. Actually, persons who reduce their carbohydrate intake usually take in less calories, since they eat less when their diet is high in fat. To build superior health on a reducing diet, however, both fat and carbohydrate must be reduced. If you eliminate refined and processed foods, your calorie intake won't be very high, even with generous amounts of natural foods.

You can raise the calorie content of your diet—without increasing your carbohydrate intake—by eating more meat, fish, and poultry. Fruits, vegetables, cereals, and bread are fairly rich in carbohydrate, but they are essential in a balanced diet. And if they are fresh and natural, you can probably handle up to 100 grams of carbohydrate and still lose weight on a moderately low-calorie diet.

HOW TO GUARD AGAINST HYPOGLYCEMIA

I've mentioned many times throughout this book that use of refined sugar and processed carbohydrates can contribute to overweight far beyond the simple addition of calories. The empty calories are bad enough; their effect on your blood sugar and your fat stores is worse. The rapid absorption of refined sugar or carbohydrate elevates the blood sugar so suddenly that a flood of insulin from the pancreas results in the storage of an excessive amount of blood sugar as glycogen, which may then be converted into fat. This means that if you eat a couple of doughnuts containing 390 calories, an insulin reaction may remove much more sugar from the blood than the doughnuts contain. Weakness, trembling, sweating, hunger, and other symptoms may then occur. This leads to a craving for sugar, which results in a progressive build-up of body fat.

How Pamela T. Controlled Her Blood Sugar with
My 10-Point Guide

I shall never forget the plight of Pamela T., an overweight nurse's aide who was so fat that people stared and snickered whenever she walked down the street. Since Pamela was young and single, she suffered all the agonies of a lonely young woman who craved the attention and companionship of a man. "I get so depressed that I frequently cry when I'm alone," she confessed. "If I could get rid of all this fat, I believe I would have more friends. I would at least have more self-confidence. But I get so weak and hungry during the day that I simply cannot pass up a doughnut or a piece of candy."

I explained to Pamela how snacking on refined and processed foods could deprive her of energy while building up body fat. I gave her a copy of the 10-point guide outlined at the end of this chapter and told her to follow it for awhile. After a couple of days, she began to eat less—and she had more energy. After a couple of weeks, she began losing weight, and by the end of the first month she was losing three or four pounds a week. I didn't recognize Pamela when I saw her six months later. She was walking through a park with a young man who was obviously interested in her. The look on her face left no doubt that she was pleased with her new self.

How to Control Your Blood Sugar with Natural Foods

The health-building natural foods reducing diet I recommend provides automatic protection against hypoglycemia. A balanced diet of natural foods supplies all the nutrients your body needs to balance metabolic processes and assure proper utilization of blood sugar and fat. Simply eliminating foods containing sugar or white flour will correct most cases of hypoglycemia. A high-protein diet, divided into five meals a day, helps maintain a consistent blood sugar level. Your diet should contain 120 to 150 grams of protein (twice as much as the average daily requirement) with 75 to 100 grams of natural carbohydrate

Your body stores a certain amount of blood sugar as glycogen, which you can draw upon when you fast or exercise. Most glycogen stores will last about two days. This is why the average person can miss a meal or two without any adverse effects. Most cases of hypoglycemia are not the result of missing a meal or a sugar-deficient diet—just the opposite. Persons suffering from hypoglycemia experience a fall in blood sugar three to five hours *after eating* a meal containing sugar or refined carbohydrate.

If you follow the basic guidelines of my fat-disintegrator diet, it's not likely that you'll have any trouble with your blood sugar. Once your bodyweight has been reduced to a desired level, remember that an "occasional" snack of refined or processed foods may be enough to throw your whole system out of balance, making it difficult to keep your blood sugar under control. So if you want to stay slim, eat natural foods—and stick to them!

How to Rule Out Organic Disease as a Cause of Hypoglycemia

If symptoms of hypoglycemia should persist in spite of frequent high-protein meals that exclude refined carbohydrates, see your doctor so that he can check you for a possible tumor on your pancreas and for adrenal cortex insufficiency.

Persons suffering from hypoglycemia caused by organic disease will usually experience weakness, trembling, hunger, and other symptoms early in the morning *before* eating breakfast. If you can't miss a meal without experiencing some of the symptoms of low blood sugar, ask your doctor for a complete medical checkup.

A 10-Point Guide for Victims of Hypoglycemia

If you suspect that you have a blood sugar problem, and you don't want to undergo a five-hour glucose tolerance test for a positive diagnosis, you can go ahead and try my 10-point guide. If it doesn't help, you may then make an appointment with your doctor. If he finds that your hypoglycemia is organic rather than functional, you'll have to remain under his care and follow his instructions.

My guide for controlling functional hypoglycemia is also effective in reducing bodyweight, and it can be used by anyone. So don't hesitate to try it.

(1) Eliminate all foods containing sugar or white flour.

(2) Do not eat processed or packaged foods. Stick strictly to natural foods.

(3) Include generous servings of meat, fish, poultry, eggs, or cheese in each meal.

(4) Select low-carbohydrate fruits and vegetables (see Chapter 3).

(5) Go easy on bread, cereals, and potatoes.

(6) Limit milk to one pint per day in order to cut down on milk sugar. Eat more fermented milk products, such as yogurt and uncreamed cottage cheese.

(7) Use cold-pressed vegetable oil on green salads in order to supply the essential fatty acids you need for a balanced metabolic process.

(8) Divide your food intake into five meals a day, or have between-meal snacks of a high-protein food such as cottage cheese or baked chicken.

(9) Carry a handful of raw nuts or toasted soybeans in your pocket in case you need an emergency snack to relieve symptoms of hypoglycemia.

(10) Steer clear of coffee, tea, colas, cigarettes, and other stimulants that may trigger hypoglycemia by stimulating your adrenal glands.

SUMMARY

1. An occasional two-day fruit-and-vegetable fast, preceded by a week of gradual reduction of food intake, will help you eat less by shrinking your stomach.

2. Eating raw fruits and vegetables during a "fast" will neutralize acids in your system and clean out your intestinal tract.

3. The average person needs about 100 grams of carbohydrate a day, but some reducing experts believe that this must be reduced to less than 75 in order to lose weight.

4. When you are counting the number of calories and the grams of carbohydrate in your diet, try to keep calories down around 1,600 and carbohydrate down around 75.

5. Remember, however, that to maintain a certain weight you must take in about 15 calories per pound of bodyweight.

6. You can raise the calorie content of your diet without increasing your carbohydrate intake simply by eating more meat, fish, or poultry.

7. No matter what type of diet you're on, you should stick to fresh, natural foods.

8. Persons who suffer from hypoglycemia or who want to lose weight should *abstain completely* from foods containing sugar or white flour and avoid processed or refined foods of any kind.

9. The type of diet used to prevent fluctuations in blood sugar will fit in well with a reducing diet.

10. When weakness, trembling, hunger, and obesity persist in spite of a sensible natural-foods diet, see your doctor for a checkup.

7

How to Fight Fat
with Normal Physical Activities

If you enjoy eating and you find it difficult to cut down the size of your meals, you can eat more and still lose weight if you'll burn a few more calories by using your muscles. Studies at Harvard University revealed that students who exercised could *double* their food intake—to about 6,000 calories a day—without gaining weight! You don't actually have to do push-ups or go to a gymnasium to get adequate exercise, however. A small amount of *normal physical activity* in combination with my fat-disintegrator diet will result in a loss of several pounds a week.

RECREATIONAL ACTIVITIES ARE BEST!

There are many ways to burn calories without doing calisthenics or lifting weights. Such recreational activities as swimming or tennis, for example, can be a pleasure rather than a chore. When you *enjoy* a physical activity, you'll push harder and play longer. And chances are you'll participate every time you have an opportunity to do so. Regular sexual activity also requires energy. If you're not an athlete or a lover, you might prefer to work off your fat doing housework, yard work, or gardening. Normal physical activities can add pleasure to a reducing program, and they can improve your health and prolong your life as well as reward you with a sense of accomplishment.

This chapter will tell you how to use up excess calories and how to burn off excess body fat with such normal, everyday activities as walking.

If you have a strenuous job and you have gained weight in spite of burning many calories, you are simply eating too much. A change in your diet is the only solution. If you are a sedentary person, however, and you get no exercise at all, a *small amount* of physical activity each day may be all that's needed to reduce your bodyweight.

Combining dietary and physical measures is the safest way to lose weight *rapidly*. Without some form of physical activity, rapid weight loss would require a low-calorie diet that might be deficient in vitamins and minerals. So if you want to lose more than three or four pounds a week, you should include a little physical activity with a balanced diet of natural foods.

How Jesse D. Trimmed Down for Marriage

Jesse D. was losing about two pounds a week on a generous diet of natural foods. He was still about 25 pounds overweight when he expressed a desire to lose more rapidly. "I'm getting married in about six weeks," he said, "and I'd like to get rid of this stomach before I go on my honeymoon."

I knew that Jesse could not tolerate a low-calorie diet, and he could certainly use a little extra strength. So I advised him to walk every chance he got and to spend at least 30 minutes each day in some form of recreational exercise. Jesse chose to swim, ride a bicycle, and play alone on an outdoor basketball court. He simply alternated these activities, depending upon how he felt. After the first week, he began to lose four or five pounds a week. He lost 26 pounds in six weeks.

"Thanks for the advice, Doc," Jesse said the day before his marriage. "I'm in great shape, and I feel fine. My wife is going to love my new body!"

IMPROVE YOUR PHYSICAL APPEARANCE WITH BETTER MUSCLE TONE

In addition to burning off ugly fat, regular physical activity will tone your muscles so that your body will be more shapely. When your muscles are firm and tight, you can carry more body fat without appearing to be fat. The contours of well-developed muscles will mold body fat into smooth, round curves. When muscles are loose and flabby, even a normal amount of body fat will sag grotesquely. Without good muscle tone, you'd have to be *skinny* to avoid a sagging anatomy—and nobody wants to be skinny. So you must have a certain amount of body fat to be physically attractive. And you must have considerable muscle to be shapely.

NORMAL PHYSICAL ACTIVITIES ALSO IMPROVE HEALTH

If you're not particularly interested in your physical appearance, remember that you *must* have some form of regular exercise to aid your heart in the circulation of blood. And the older you become, the more important it is to aid the circulation of blood with muscle contraction. Exercise will strengthen your heart and your bones as well as your muscles, giving you the reserve strength you need to meet unexpected physical emergencies.

If you want to live life fully, you'll need the extra strength and endurance that comes from regular physical activity. It's no fun to complete each day on the brink of exhaustion because you are so physically unfit that simple sitting becomes work. Besides, persons who sit or lie down many hours each day without getting any exercise at all often develop circulatory problems and blood clots that can lead to a heart attack or loss of a leg. *So whether you are overweight or not, you should entertain yourself each day with some form of recreational activity that uses your muscles.*

Swimming, bicycle riding, and similar activities are actually *fun*. Treat yourself and take time out from your busy schedule for a little outdoor activity. You'll lose your excess body fat much more rapidly—and you'll feel better and live longer.

"I'm Too Tired. . ."

Many inactive people complain that they are "too tired" to walk, ride a bicycle, or rake the yard. Actually, they are tired *because* of their inactivity. Flabby muscles, poor circulation, and a sluggish metabolic process barely produce enough energy to sustain life. As a result, practically all of the calories consumed are stored as fat. With no physical activity to switch on the metabolic processes that control energy intake and output, an uncontrolled appetite simply builds up body fat.

There is some evidence to indicate that the average sedentary person eats *more* than an active person. There is no reason to believe that normal physical activity will stimulate the appetite. Quite the contrary. Practically all obese people are less active than lean people. Combine inactivity with a large appetite and obesity is unavoidable.

When a person gets some form of regular exercise in normal physical activities, calorie intake is usually equal to calorie output. This keeps the weight normal and constant. Nature has a way of *controlling* the appetite when the muscles are conditioned by regular exercise. Bodyweight is normalized when the appetite mechanism is governed by an active and wide-awake body.

DISPOSE OF EXCESS CALORIES WITH A TUNED-UP METABOLISM

After you have been on a reducing diet for a few months and you have lost a considerable amount of weight, weight loss will be slower because your body learns to function more efficiently on fewer calories. When this happens, some form of regular physical activity will result in additional weight **loss**.

Considering all the benefits of regular exercise, it would be much better to spend a few calories in physical activity rather than restrict your diet too severely. Chances are your bodyweight will normalize on a prolonged natural foods diet. But if you do have difficulty losing the last few pounds, or if you want to *speed* weight loss, you can't go wrong with a little exercise.

Once your body has been conditioned by regular physical activity, your metabolic process will dispose of excess calories even when you aren't exercising. This means that when you're "in shape" you won't have to "work off" every extra calorie you take in, and you'll be able to eat more without gaining weight.

How Much Exercise Do You Need?

Most conditioning experts agree that the average middle-aged person should spend at least 30 minutes a day in some physical activity that burns 300 or more calories—or about 10 calories a minute. It isn't necessary, however, to get all your exercise in one marathon session. *Frequent periods of a small amount of exercise may be more effective in reducing bodyweight than one long period.*

You certainly do not want to push yourself to the point of pain or exhaustion. If you have a room to paint, for example, you might actually enjoy painting one wall a day rather than attempt to paint the entire room at one time. You'll do a better job as well as get more exercise.

HOW TO GET PLENTY OF EXERCISE WITHOUT EXERCISING

There are many normal, everyday activities that you can work into your daily routine for reducing purposes. When your yard needs raking, for example, do it yourself rather than hire someone for the job. Working in the yard will tone your muscles, stimulate your circulation, clean out your lungs with fresh air, and expose your skin to sunlight.

Walking to the store or riding a bicycle to work will provide an "easy" form of exercise that can be repeated many times during the week. Such simple activities as walking can make your reducing diet much more effective. When overweight students at the University of Minnesota were placed on a 1,200 calorie diet, those who walked lost more weight. "Students who had no special exercise program lost an average of three pounds a week; those who walked averaged a loss of five pounds a week, improved their fitness, and suffered no more from hunger pangs than did the nonexercisers."

Select Your Own Calorie-Burning Activity

It's not likely that you'll often participate in an activity that's strenuous enough to burn 10 calories a minute, as suggested by some fitness experts. But if you select something you *enjoy* doing and participate *often,* you'll burn enough calories to take care of the excess. Remember that in the long run you'll burn *more* calories in frequent, short bouts of exercise than in an occasional intense effort. So don't be concerned about how many calories you're burning a minute. Just concentrate on making a prolonged *comfortable* effort. *Stop* when you begin to experience discomfort of any type. Resume the activity when you feel energetic enough to do so.

HOW TO MEASURE YOUR EXERCISE

In order to judge the effect of the exercise you get in normal physical activities, you'll have to have some idea of the number of calories you're burning. Gardening and recreational swimming, for example, burn about five calories a minute. One hour of brisk walking uses about 480 calories. Climbing stairs burns about seven calories a minute. Canoeing, bicycling, dancing the rumba, and tennis require about seven calories a minute. Simply digging a hole in the garden uses about 8.5 calories a minute. Dancing the twist requires as many as 10 calories a minute, or about the same as cross-country running. (This may explain the quick demise of the twist!)

Moderate exercise burns five to seven calories a minute. *Strenuous* exercise burns 10 or more calories a minute.

Condition Yourself Gradually

Some forms of recreational exercise can be just as strenuous as push-ups and other forms of exercise. The difference is that you *enjoy* the recreational exercise, so you don't mind it. You'll have to be careful, therefore, not to overdo it when you begin a physical activity for the first time. Always begin lightly and slowly work your way up to a full or prolonged effort. If you want to start a garden, for example, you shouldn't spend too much time on the project the first day. You may become so sore that you'll give up the project altogether. Start digging early enough to give yourself plenty of time to get ready for the planting season.

Remember that it takes about six weeks to become fully conditioned for a strenuous physical activity. So don't rush! If the activity you select seems to be too strenuous for you, just do a little at a time. Chances are you'll lose more weight if you'll spread out your activity than you would in 30 minutes of continuous activity.

BRISK WALKING IS IDEAL FOR MOST FOLKS

Any form of physical activity that uses the big muscles of your thighs will burn calories and condition your body. So whenever possible, *use your legs!* Walking is a convenient form of physical activity for most of us. Walking can also be useful in shopping, visiting, and working. Resolve *now* to walk as much as possible as often as possible. When you go shopping, park your car a few blocks away from your destination and then walk the rest of the way. When you have a choice, use the stairs instead of the elevator. If the neighborhood grocery store is not too far away, walk to the store *every day* to purchase fresh meats and vegetables. (Remember that it's best to cook fresh vegetables each day rather than eat leftovers if you want maximum nutrition with minimum calories on a fat-disintegrator diet. Walking to the grocery store will burn calories as well as keep you supplied with nourishing, low-calorie foods.)

How to Walk Properly

When you first begin walking, walk slowly for a short distance the first few days. Then gradually increase the speed and distance. Rapid walking for a couple of blocks will strengthen your heart as well as burn calories. The faster you walk the more calories you'll burn, but remember that it's better to walk frequently and comfortably than to push yourself uncomfortably for a short period of time. If you'll simply work walking into your daily activities, you'll get all the exercise you need without really exercising.

Most of us walk about 2.5 miles an hour. When you walk for physical fitness, however, you should walk about four miles an hour—or twice as fast as normal. This will increase the burning of calories from about three a minute to five a minute. If you live in a big city, you may be able to walk to work faster than you can drive. Traffic in New York City, for example, moves about three to four miles an hour. You can *walk* faster than that! Park your car and walk when the traffic is heavy. It'll be easier on your nervous system, better for your heart, and a big help in reducing your bodyweight.

Note: If you have foot trouble and cannot walk much, exercise your legs by riding a bicycle or by swimming. Any exercise that uses the big muscles of your thighs will burn a large number of calories.

HOW TO TEST THE EFFECTIVENESS OF PHYSICAL ACTIVITY

Combining diet and exercise should result in a loss of four or five pounds a week, which is enough if you want to eat generously and maintain the best of health. The more exercise you take, the more weight you'll lose and the more physically fit you'll become.

You can test your physical fitness simply by taking your pulse rate. If it is high, or above 80, your heart is beating too fast because it is weak or because your body does not function efficiently. Take your pulse in a sitting position and record the figure on a piece of paper. After you have been physically active for several weeks, check your pulse again. It should be considerably lower. The lower your pulse, the better your physical condition and the less strain there is on your heart and lungs. (Take your pulse before you eat so that it won't be elevated by a full stomach.)

As you become better conditioned physically, you can do more with less discomfort. Until you have spent several weeks conditioning your body, however, don't go "all out" in any physical activity. If you swim, play tennis, or participate in some other enjoyable recreational activity, the exercise may be so invigorating that you'll be tempted to push yourself until you "give out." Don't do it! Remember that you can burn more calories by being moderately active throughout the day than by endangering yourself with overexertion.

COMBINE DEEP BREATHING WITH NORMAL PHYSICAL ACTIVITIES

Always breathe deeply when you get a little breathless from physical exertion. Lifting your chest during inhalation will actually aid the circulation of blood by placing a suction effect on the large veins that drain your lower body.

Of course, it's always a good idea to take an occasional deep breath to clean out the remote air sacs in your lungs. But forced deep breathing when you don't need the extra oxygen will upset the chemical balance of your blood by "blowing off" too much carbon dioxide. This will constrict the blood vessels around your brain, resulting in dizziness caused by a slowdown in circulation. Always stop forced deep breathing when you begin to feel dizzy or light-headed.

RELIEVE TENSION WITH PHYSICAL ACTIVITY

Normal physical activities throughout the day will provide calorie-burning exercise that you won't think of as being "exercise." When you do want to exercise strenuously, it's best to do so at the end of the day *before your evening meal.* You should never exercise with a full stomach. If you can't use your muscles before you eat, wait at least two hours after eating before you exert yourself.

Exercise relieves tension, relaxes muscles, and works off the day's frustrations. If you take a moderate amount of exercise before you sit down for your evening meal, you'll be relaxed enough to enjoy eating. Follow your meal with a warm bath and you'll be ready for a good night's sleep.

Note: Although exercise taken before the evening meal relieves tension, an excessive amount of exercise taken just before bedtime may result in insomnia caused by "wide awake nerves."

WATCH THE WEATHER!

If you choose to exercise strenuously because of the challenge it offers or because you enjoy exercising, be careful not to push yourself too hard during extremely hot or cold weather. Do not exercise when the temperature is higher than 85 degrees Fahrenheit or lower than 40 degrees, or when the relative humidity is more than 80 percent.

Finish your exercise with a short walk to keep your blood circulating while you recover from the exercise. If you exercise strenuously for several minutes and then suddenly stand still, dizziness or fainting may occur from a sudden slowdown in circulation.

WATCH OUT FOR CHEST AND LEG PAIN

Whatever type of physical activity you choose to use to burn excess calories, remember that you should begin lightly and slowly increase the amount of work you do. This will give your muscles time to become accustomed to the effort, and it will protect your heart from strain. As your muscles become stronger, your heart will also become stronger. Always discontinue an exertion, however, if you begin to experience chest or leg pain. If you happen to have hardened or clogged arteries, you might feel chest and arm pain from lack of adequate blood flow to your heart when it is beating rapidly. Or you might suffer from leg cramps caused by poor circulation to the muscles of your calves.

In either case, you should see your doctor for a checkup. Most of the time, your doctor will advise you to continue with your physical activity in order to open up the narrow blood vessels. Just remember to stop and rest when you feel chest, arm, neck, or leg pain. Each time you exercise, however, you should be able to do a little more without feeling the pain.

INCREASE YOUR STAMINA WITH VITAMIN E AND WHEAT GERM OIL

A couple tablespoons of wheat germ oil added to your fat-disintegrator diet, as recommended in Chapter 3, will supply Vitamin E that will help open clogged arteries. The essential fatty acids in the oil will aid in the disintegration of hard fat in your body. Studies at the University of Illinois have shown that a substance in wheat germ oil (other than Vitamin E) will also increase stamina and endurance. A group of middle-aged men who took one teaspoonful of wheat germ oil daily while training on a treadmill had 51 percent more endurance than a group that trained without taking the oil. This added endurance will help you burn far more calories than the oil supplies.

You may take a Vitamin E supplement along with wheat germ oil. Try taking about 300 units of Vitamin E daily or 100 units with each meal.

WHAT ABOUT SPOT REDUCING?

Flabby buttocks and sagging breasts are common among persons who get no exercise at all. Even when an individual is not overweight, flabby muscles may allow fatty tissue in the breasts and buttocks to sag. A small amount of exercise to tighten and firm-up the supporting muscles will help restore firm, attractive contours.

You cannot "spot reduce" an isolated area of the body with exercise or diet. When you exercise the muscles underlying fatty tissue, improved muscle tone will improve the shape of the exercised area, but calories burned in performance of the exercise will result in an *overall* weight loss.

SIMPLE EXERCISES TO IMPROVE THE SHAPE OF HIPS AND BREASTS

Here are a few specific exercises you can use to shape up your hips and your breasts. Once you have become accustomed to doing these exercises, you can do them in rapid repetitions to burn calories as well as to tone your muscles.

1. *The supine lateral raise:* Lie on your back on the floor. Hold a light weight in each hand at arm's length over your chest. Keep your arms straight and inhale deeply while lowering the weights to the floor on each side. Return to starting position and repeat. (See Figure 1.)

Occasionally lower the weight back over your head (to the floor) with straight arms, inhaling deeply as the weight goes back.

Use a weight in each hand that you can handle for several repetitions without strain. About ten pounds in each hand will be about right for most people.

The supine lateral raise will tone up the muscles underlying your breasts and improve their shape.

2. *Modified push-ups:* Push-ups (with your knees on the floor) can be substituted effectively for supine lateral raises. Try to do at least six repetitions. This exercise will tighten up the muscles on the back of your arms as well as improve the shape of your chest. (See Figure 2.)

3. *The flat-footed squat:* Hold on to a bedpost for balance and do a full squat. *Keep both feet flat on the floor while you squat.* Keep your head up and your upper body as erect as possible. (See Figure 3.)

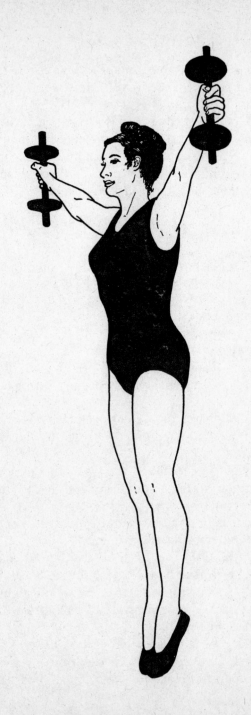

Figure 1: Supine Lateral Raise

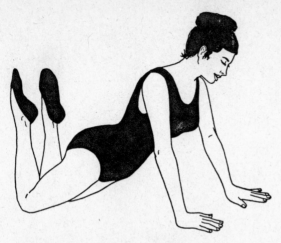

Figure 2: Modified Push-Ups

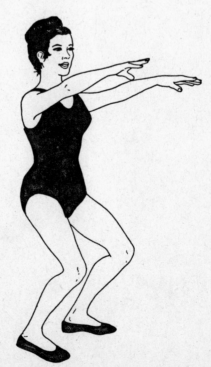

Figure 3: Flat-Footed Squat

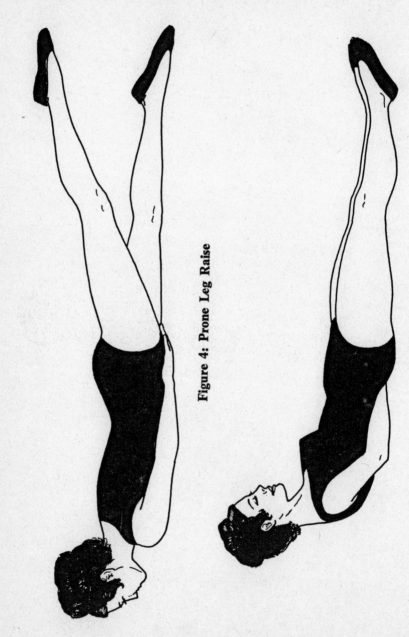

Figure 4: Prone Leg Raise

Figure 5: Trunk Curl

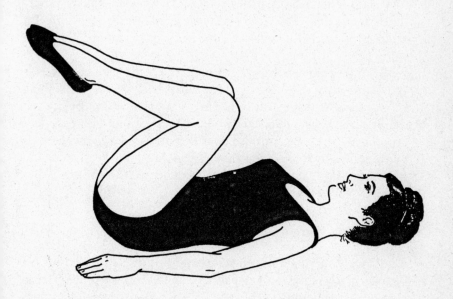

Figure 6: Knee-to-Chest Leg Raise

A flat-footed squat is probably the best exercise you can do for the muscles of your hips. Do five or six squats every time you get an opportunity. You should eventually be able to do the exercise without holding on to a bedpost.

Note: There is less strain on your knees when you do a flat-footed squat than when you squat on your toes. If you do feel a strain on your knees, however, do a half squat rather than a full squat.

4. *Prone leg raise:* If you cannot squat, do this exercise for your buttock muscles. Lie face down and raise one leg as high as you can. Keep the leg as straight as possible. (See Figure 4.) Exercise both legs alternately, about 10 repetitions with each leg.

Since the prone leg raise does not use the large muscles on the front of your thighs, you should also do squats if you possibly can. Squatting exercises burn calories as well as improve the shape of your thighs and hips.

What About Your Abdomen?

If your abdomen sags because of loose or flabby abdominal muscles, a simple "stomach exercise" will improve your physical appearance and reduce the size of your waistline. Remember, however, that abdominal exercises will not "spot reduce" your abdomen. Any exercise that burns calories will reduce fat all over your body. The normal physical activities recommended earlier in this chapter will be more effective than "stomach exercises" in burning the fat off your abdomen.

5. *Trunk curl:* Lie on your back on the floor and curl your head and shoulders up from the floor. Concentrate on contracting your abdominal muscles. It isn't necessary to do a complete sit-up. Keep your lower back on the floor and do as many trunk curls as necessary to fatigue your abdominal muscles. (See Figure 5.)

6. *Knee-to-chest leg raise:* Lie flat on the floor with your legs straight and your arms alongside your body. Raise your legs (while bending your knees) and try to touch your knees to your chin. Try to do at least 10 repetitions. (See Figure 6.)

YOU CAN'T MASSAGE OR "BUMP OFF" FATTY TISSUE

Many people believe that massage, vibrators, and pounding will dispose of fatty tissue by "breaking it up." Vibrator belts and rollers are still popular in gyms and health clubs, and it's not at all uncommon to hear of women who bump their hips against a wall in order to "break down the fat."

Actually, the only way fat can be removed from the body is to *burn* it off in the body's metabolic fires. You can accomplish this by controlling your diet or by exercising your muscles so that you burn more calories each day than you take in. Of course, the best approach is to combine dietary measures with a moderate amount of physical activity so that you can eat generously and avoid strenuous exercise.

You can eventually lose all of your excess body fat with my natural foods fat-disintegrator diet, but weight loss will be more rapid and your health will be better if you burn a little fat with exercise.

In any event, don't waste time and money trying to massage away fat. It would be better to make love or go dancing.

REDUCE WITH SEX!

Any kind of physical activity will help regulate your bodyweight by tuning the mechanism that controls your body's use of calories. Since sexual intercourse requires a considerable amount of energy, you can include sexual activities in your program of normal activities for reducing purposes.

If you read my book *Doctor Homola's Life-Extender Health Guide,* you know that regular sexual activity helps prolong your life by improving your health.

For greater pleasure and a slimmer body, think of sex as a form of exercise that can be as beneficial as walking or working in the garden.

STAY PHYSICALLY ACTIVE!

It really does not matter what type of physical activity you use to burn calories as long as it keeps you active. Obviously, it would be best to participate in a *variety* of activities each day.

Recreational and constructive activities, such as bicycle riding and yard work, won't be boring or excessively tiring.

If you dread an activity, chances are you'll find some excuse to avoid it. There are plenty of normal activities—from walking to sex—that you can use to keep yourself physically active. Home maintenance provides many good opportunities for a little constructive exercise. Mowing your lawn, painting your house, cleaning out a storeroom, and so on, will provide an endless string of chores for you if you take pride in your home.

Remember that it's better to get your exercise in small amounts *frequently* rather than in one painful marathon session. So do a little at a time, several times a day, *every day.*

FOR WOMEN ONLY: WHAT ABOUT "CELLULITE"?

The word "cellulite" is not in my medical dictionary, and I cannot find any reference to it in my textbooks. So I don't really know much about it, except that some people use the term to describe the lumpy tissue that appears under the skin of some women. Books dealing with cellulite describe it as a form of connective tissue that cannot be disposed of by diet alone It has been my observation that "cellulite" does not appear in women who are slim and trim and who exercise regularly.

I have always felt that the lumps referred to as cellulite are simply irregular collections of fat that have probably ruptured cell walls and membranes. This fat can be burned off just like any other fat. And when the muscles are toned and enlarged with regular exercise, body fat is more evenly distributed and molded by the support of the skeletal muscles.

If you reduce your body fat with my fat-disintegrator diet and then use physical activity to shape your muscles, chances are that the lumpy fat on your body will eventually disappear. If you'll trim down (and develop your muscles) so that you cannot pinch up more than an inch of fat on your upper arm, the ruptured and scarred fat cells probably won't bulge.

Since women normally have a thick layer of fatty tissue covering their body, they naturally have more trouble with lumpy fat than men do. If this layer of fat is allowed to get too thick, the beautiful, round feminine curves are transformed into sagging, lumpy flesh. And without adequate muscle to mold the overlying fatty tissue, the body no longer has the shape that is so appealing to the eye.

It's entirely possible that once fat cells have ruptured the surrounding membranes, a certain amount of lumpiness may be permanent. Reduction of fat, however, along with development of the muscles should result in great improvement.

Cellulite Is Not the Same as Cellulitis

Bulging lumps of ruptured fat cells are not to be confused with painful fibrous deposits that are composed primarily of connective tissue. I find these deposits frequently in the muscles and tissues of sedentary persons who do not receive enough circulatory stimulation to flush out toxic wastes. Moist heat, massage, and exercise will eventually "work out" fibrous deposits, but fat deposits must be burned as energy.

Connective tissue in the body can become inflamed and cause cellulitis, which is a painful condition that is not related to the lumpy fat deposits called "cellulite."

10 Ways to Combat Cellulite

If there is such a thing as cellulite, the scar tissue that traps fat, water, and toxic wastes in compartments beneath the skin might respond to these measures:

1. Regular exercise to burn calories and develop muscles.
2. Moist heat and massage to stimulate circulation and to soften connective tissue.
3. A low-calorie diet of natural foods, combined with regular physical activity to *force* burning of stored body fat.
4. Since lumpy deposits of fatty tissue are often associated with hormonal changes in women, 200 to 400 units of Vitamin E each day might be of value in preventing the development of cellulite.

5. Reduction of the amount of salt in the diet might help prevent retention of water in fatty tissue.

6. A good, balanced diet, such as that recommended in Chapter 2, will prevent the nutritional deficiencies that might contribute to rupturing and scarring of fat cells and tissue membranes. Vitamins A and C, for example, will strengthen the collagen that holds tissue cells together.

7. If you're not already fat, avoid getting fat so that you won't stretch connective tissue with expanding fat cells.

8. Do the exercises described in this chapter in order to develop the muscles in your thighs and buttocks.

9. Occasionally cover your body with a little vegetable oil (or a Vitamin E cream) and give yourself a massage. Rub the lumpy areas vigorously, always rubbing toward your heart.

10. A moderate sun tan will help conceal lumpy flesh by improving skin tone.

SURGICAL REMOVAL OF "FAT PADS"

Some people inherit unsightly fatty tissue deposits, or "fat pads," that cannot be removed except by starvation or by surgery. If you have such a pad under your chin, on the back of your arms, on your hips, or on some other visible spot, you might consider consulting a plastic surgeon.

Most men prefer that a woman's body be well padded rather than skinny. So don't try to get rid of an isolated fat pad by starving your entire body until it is bony and stringy. Remember that female pulchritude depends largely upon fatty tissue that is molded by well-developed muscles. Every woman needs a little fat to be soft and cuddly. And she needs a little muscle to be shapely.

How Leona K. Smoothed Her Lumpy Flesh

Leona K. had such lumpy, bulging thighs that she absolutely refused to wear shorts or a bathing suit. She was also overweight and physically weak. I put Leona on my fat-disintegrator diet and recommended the exercises described in this chapter. She lost 48 pounds of body fat in six months. The exercises she took for her thighs and buttocks enlarged the muscles enough to smooth out the overlying fatty tissue. Development of Leona's thigh muscles made her much more attractive by giving her thighs and buttocks a full, round appearance.

"I used to be reluctant to let my husband see my thighs," Leona confessed. "But I look so much better since I started your diet and exercise program that I'm now quite proud of my physical appearance. In fact, I just purchased my first bikini bathing suit, and with the full approval of my husband. Thanks for all your help and advice."

Leona was, indeed, an eyeful. And seeing the change in her body and in her mental attitude was reward enough for the effort I made on her behalf.

SUMMARY

1. Research indicates that you can eat twice as much without gaining weight or lose twice as much weight on a restricted diet if you include a small amount of daily exercise.

2. You can get all the exercise you need with normal physical activities that use your muscles in a pleasant and constructive manner.

3. In addition to burning calories, aiding the circulation of blood, and strengthening your heart, regular exercise will improve your physical appearance by shaping the muscles of your body.

4. When the body is conditioned by regular exercise in normal physical activities, bodyweight is automatically normalized by a balance in calorie intake and output.

5. Frequent, comfortable physical activity is much more beneficial for reducing purposes than one prolonged exertion.

6. Lumpy fat known as cellulite can usually be eliminated by reducing body fat and developing the skeletal muscles.

7. Activities that involve use of the big muscles of the thighs are best for burning calories and conditioning the body.

8. When you are "tired" and tense, exercise provided by recreational activity will rejuvenate you as well as dispose of excess calories.

9. Good news! Regular sexual activity can be considered a form of normal physical activity that burns calories.

10. It really does not matter how you use your muscles to burn calories as long as you *stay physically active.*

8

How to Switch
from a Fat-Disintegrator Diet
to a Fat-Fighting Diet

Most reducing diets are so restrictive or so skimpy that the suffering dieter can hardly wait to quit the diet and start eating "normally." This is exactly why so many reducing diets fail—because the diets can be followed on a short-term basis only. Then, when the dieter begins to resume his old eating habits, he quickly regains lost weight.

On my natural foods fat-disintegrator diet, you make a *permanent change* in your eating habits. You learn how to select and prepare natural foods that you can eat every day of your life. With no fancy foods to artificially stimulate your appetite, you'll automatically eat the correct amount of food, and your bodyweight will normalize itself. With a few simple tricks, such as an occasional two-day fast, frequent small meals, special cooking methods, and regular physical activity, you can satisfy your appetite and still lose weight.

The best feature of my fat-disintegrator diet is that even when your weight is down to normal you can continue the diet without fear of losing any more weight. The reason for this is that when you eat *properly,* both your appetite and your bodyweight will automatically adjust to what is best for *you.*

Once your weight is down to where it should be, you might be tempted to relax your guard over what you eat. If you do, be sure to weigh yourself at least once a week. When you discover that you are two or three pounds above your ideal weight, eliminate the forbidden foods and increase your physical activity.

THE FIRST RULE OF DIETING STILL APPLIES

Remember that no matter how slim you might become, it's *never* a good idea to eat refined and processed foods. In addition to containing empty calories, processed foods often contain harmful preservatives and artificial additives. So when I refer to "forbidden foods" in my fat-fighting diet, I mean potatoes with butter, meat fat, breads, cereals, high-carbohydrate vegetables, natural ice cream, and other calorie-rich or high-carbohydrate natural foods that must be eaten sparingly in a reducing diet.

When my wife bakes whole-wheat bread, it is very tempting for me to sit down and eat half a loaf of the warm bread (especially with butter). I exercise my willpower, however, and eat only one slice of the delicious bread. You can use your willpower, too, in limiting your consumption of delicious but fattening foods. Just remember that you're choosing between temporarily satisfying your taste buds or maintaining a permanently attractive body.

Continue with Natural Foods

Many people will not gain weight eating natural foods. Others may find it necessary to go easy on certain high-calorie natural foods. It's entirely possible that once your weight has been reduced with a fat-disintegrator diet you might be able to eat generously of any natural food without gaining weight. The reason for this is that all of your overweight originally came from refined and processed foods that do nothing but build up body fat. Simply switching from refined foods to natural foods may be all you need to do to lose excess body fat. Once this switch is made, no further changes may be necessary. Your pancreas should eventually lose its sensitivity so that you can eat *any* natural carbohydrate without gaining weight. You may then begin to include more of your favorite high-calorie *natural* foods. In other words, you switch from a fat-disintegrator diet to a fat-fighting diet.

How Corinne P. Switched from a Fat-Disintegrator Diet to a Fat-Fighting Diet

Corinne P. stayed on my fat-disintegrator diet for only three months before switching to a fat-fighting diet. Her weight dropped from 163 to 115, a loss of 48 pounds. "I love fried chicken and homemade ice cream," Corinne confessed. "Would it be all right to fry my chicken occasionally? I have a lot of company, and I'd like to serve them some of my special peach ice cream."

Since Corinne had lost so much weight so rapidly, I told her to go ahead and try eating a little fried chicken and natural ice cream once a week and see what happened. She did not gain an ounce over the next four weeks! Since her weight had already normalized, she stayed about the same—no gain and no loss.

It could be that you, too, will be able to increase the calorie content of your diet (with natural foods) without regaining lost weight, provided you follow the instructions outlined in this chapter. Once you have *conquered* fat, you should have no trouble *fighting* fat.

USE THE MIRROR CHECK

In Chapter 3, I suggested that you view your nude body in a mirror to judge the amount of fat you have. After you are slim and trim, you should continue to use the mirror to check for signs of a build-up of body fat. Carry a slim image in your mind so that you'll be psychologically conditioned for a constant awareness of what you eat. Think of all the advantages a slim person has in buying clothes, winning friends, and making love. A little attention to what you eat is a small price to pay for all the benefits of a lean, healthy body.

TREAT YOURSELF OCCASIONALLY WITH
FRIED CHICKEN OR FISH

When you were in the process of reducing your weight, you were advised to eat baked or broiled chicken, fish, and lean meat that had all the visible fat cut away. You should continue eating fish, poultry, and lean meat, but it might be all right to occasionally eat a little fried chicken or fish if no batter is used and if all the grease is drained away on paper towels while the food is still hot. Be sure to peel the skin of chicken away, however, before cooking or before eating. Practically all of the fat of poultry is in the skin.

When fish or chicken has been fried, you should eat *less* than you would if it were broiled or baked. This may be difficult to do, since fried foods are often more tasty than broiled foods.

Fish has more protein and fewer calories than meat. So eat fish as often as possible, preferably broiled.

ENJOY THE TASTE OF WHOLE MILK

Skimmed milk and uncreamed cottage cheese are good sources of low-fat protein for a fat-disintegrator diet, but once your weight is down you may occasionally have whole milk and a little of your favorite yellow cheese (for taste as well as for the Vitamin A they supply). Remember, however, that you must go easy on any kind of animal fat if you want to protect your arteries. So even if you find that whole milk and cheese do not seem to increase your weight, you must use them sparingly or only on special occasions.

You should *never* eat processed cheese, no matter how thin you might be. A fat-fighting diet should also be a health-building diet. And this means sticking strictly to *natural* foods. Processed foods usually contain artificial additives and are often deficient in nutrients. Don't forget that the secret of a successful reducing diet is getting a maximum amount of nutrients from a minimum amount of food. When you eat processed foods, you get maximum calories with *minimum* nutrients. So when you switch from a fat-disintegrator diet to a fat-fighting diet, it's important to continue eating natural foods.

CONTINUE EATING SALADS

Fresh, raw salads should be a part of your daily fat-fighting diet. Most of the time, you should use a dressing made of vegetable oil, vinegar, and lemon juice. You must have a small amount of vegetable oil in your diet for good health, and it's best used with salads so that it won't be damaged by heat. You may occasionally use a commercial dressing if it is made from vegetable oil and limited to two tablespoons daily. Mayonnaise, for example, is a soft vegetable fat that won't harm your arteries.

Note: Remember that oily salad dressings are high in calories and must be used sparingly. If you use vegetable oil, do not use mayonnaise, and vice versa. A tablespoonful of salad oil contains about 124 calories, a tablespoonful of mayonnaise about 93 calories. Both can be diluted with vinegar or lemon juice for use in a large salad.

WIDEN YOUR CHOICE OF VEGETABLES

When you are on a fat-disintegrator diet, you must go easy on certain high-carbohydrate vegetables. On a fat-fighting diet, however, you may eat reasonable portions of any fresh vegetable as long as it has not been cooked with oil, grease, or butter. If the vegetable has been properly cooked, that is, if it has not been overcooked, the fibers or cellulose in the vegetable will pass through the intestinal tract undigested, thus reducing absorption of calories.

EAT GENEROUSLY!

Although some low-carbohydrate diets severely restrict the use of vegetables, I have never been convinced that properly prepared vegetables of any kind are fattening. Natural carbohydrates do not stimulate the appetite, and they are absorbed and digested more slowly than refined carbohydrates.

One of my patients, Janice T., lost 20 pounds in eight weeks on my fat-disintegrator diet. When she switched to my fat-fighting diet, she ate any amount of all the fresh vegetables she wanted. She continued to lose a pound a week until her weight leveled off at an attractive 113 pounds. Weight loss was not so rapid as on the fat-disintegrator diet, but she continued to shed *excess* fat until her weight normalized, in spite of eating generous amounts of fresh vegetables.

In order to make sure that her vegetables were always fresh, Janice started her own garden. The exercise she got taking care of the garden and the constant supply of low-calorie vegetables kept her slim and trim without any trouble at all. "I dearly love fresh vegetables," Janice declared. "I truly feel sorry for persons who starve themselves to lose weight or who literally *kill* their appetite with fatty, greasy foods."

Every time I see a suffering dieter sit down to a meal of black coffee and lettuce leaves, it's all I can do not to cry out, "Hey! You don't have to starve yourself! Why not try the broiled fish, with stringbeans and a tossed salad? Or the baked chicken with steamed cabbage and sliced tomatoes?" There are many wholesome foods that can satisfy the appetite without building up body fat.

If you apply what you learn from reading this book, you won't ever have to subject yourself to a dangerous "high-fat reducing diet" or a starvation diet. You'll know better, and you'll be knowledgeable enough to use your own judgement to plan your meals.

SUGAR-SWEETENED DRINKS ARE STILL A NO-NO

Very little change is made in the use of beverages on a fat-fighting diet, with the exception that you can use some whole milk and more unsweetened fruit juices. Remember that no matter how slim you are, you should continue to *avoid the use of sugar-sweetened drinks.*

Artificial sweeteners may be more harmful to your body than sugar. So it's best to do without sweeteners of any type, even honey.

An occasional cocktail might be all right if liberal use of natural foods does not seem to trigger an increase in weight. If you find that inclusion of high-calorie natural carbohydrate foods results in a gain in weight, however, you certainly do not need the empty calories supplied by alcohol.

FATS AND OILS SHOULD ALWAYS BE RESTRICTED

Too much animal fat, even from natural sources, can contribute to the development of hardened arteries, premature aging heart disease, cancer, and overweight. Too much oil of any type can speed the aging process and cause cancer. So there are good reasons why you should go easy on fats and oils, even after you have reduced your bodyweight. A fat-fighting diet, like a fat-disintegrator diet, should improve your health and lengthen your life as well as combat body fat.

WHAT ABOUT DESSERT?

Although I usually advise *all* of my patients to avoid sugar and white-flour products, I would not deny a slim person an occasional cookie, a small amount of ice cream, or a piece of mom's apple pie. If you continue to eat natural foods after you have reduced your bodyweight, you can probably have an "unnatural sweet" once in a while without any harmful effects, but only *after* a regular meal. I do hope, however, that you'll learn to prefer fresh and dried fruits for dessert, so that you won't be tempted to reach into a cookie jar.

If you discover that a refined or unnatural sweet triggers a gain in weight, it may mean that your pancreas is still overly sensitive. If this is the case after you have spent several weeks on a fat-disintegrator diet, it may mean that your body does not tolerate refined sweets. You may also be "allergic" to white-flour products. If so, you are a "carboholic," and you must avoid refined carbohydrates and sweets the way an alcoholic must avoid alcohol.

GO EASY ON SALT

While you are reducing your bodyweight, you should try to avoid excessive use of table salt, since salt forces your body to retain water. You can get all the salt you need from natural foods (if you do not perspire excessively). When you are slim and trim, however, you can use a little salt occasionally for a taste treat. When you live dangerously and eat a little fried chicken, for example, its taste can be greatly enhanced by a sprinkle of salt.

When you do use salt, always use the iodized variety (or get your iodine from seafood). If you use bouillon cubes in cooking, remember that regular bouillon contains salt. If you find yourself gaining weight, substitute salt-free bouillon.

Note: I do not recommend the use of monosodium glutamate as a seasoning, since it is an artificial product that may have harmful side effects. Many people who use this popular seasoning experience a variety of symptoms that doctors have labeled the "Chinese restaurant syndrome," since they were first noticed in persons who ate highly seasoned Chinese food.

WATCH YOUR WEIGHT CLOSELY

When you were on my fat-disintegrator diet, you lost weight because certain food items were restricted or prohibited. Once your weight has normalized and you no longer have any excess body fat, you might be able to sneak a few goodies occasionally without regaining lost weight. You must be totally honest with yourself, however, and you must weigh yourself frequently. When you discover that you are two or three pounds over your ideal weight, you must again restrict your diet to fat-disintegrator foods. This means that you must reduce or eliminate the high-calorie natural foods, such as bread, butter, dried fruit, potatoes, and honey, that build up body fat or overwork your pancreas. And you should again read the opening chapters of this book.

Actually, if you switch to natural foods and make permanent changes in your eating habits and then go easy on the high-calorie foods, you shouldn't have any trouble controlling your bodyweight.

To repeat: On a fat-fighting diet, you should continue to avoid refined and processed foods, especially foods containing sugar and white flour, and eat only *natural* foods. You may, however, eat more of the high-calorie natural foods if they do not trigger a gain in weight.

EXERCISE AND A FAT-FIGHTING DIET

Although diet is the best approach to use in controlling bodyweight, a small amount of exercise can do wonders in helping you keep your weight down if you want to eat high-calorie natural foods. If you begin to eat mashed potatoes with butter, for example, you can dispose of the excess calories with a little exercise.

Normal physical activity or recreational exercise, as recommended in Chapter 7, will entertain you as well as burn calories. The more exercise you get, the more you can eat without regaining lost weight. Remember, however, that if you begin to include a few high-calorie foods in your diet, you cannot increase the *volume* of food you eat. On a fat-fighting diet, as on a fat-disintegrator diet, you must choose between eating generous amounts of low-calorie foods or restricting your diet in order to include a few high-calorie foods. I personally prefer to eat generous amounts of all the basic natural foods and then go easy on the high-calorie foods so that I don't have to take an excessive amount of exercise.

Even if you are slim and not gaining weight, you should not stuff yourself or overeat. Don't think that just because you are no longer overweight you can forget about the calorie-content of foods. *The best reducing diet is a lifetime diet.* And there is some evidence to indicate that a low-calorie diet prolongs life. So don't load your diet with more calories than you can work off with a moderate amount of normal physical activity.

COUNTING CALORIES FOR WEIGHT MAINTENANCE

Although bodyweight tends to normalize when the diet is limited to natural foods, you might occasionally want to count the calories in your daily meals just to see if you're over or under the recommended number needed to maintain your ideal weight.

You'll recall from reading Chapter 6 that the average person needs about 15 calories daily per pound of bodyweight to maintain the existing weight. This means that when your weight is finally down to a certain level you must not exceed a certain number of calories each day if you do not exercise regularly. If you are an inactive person, you might not be able to exceed 12 or 13 calories per pound of bodyweight if you want to stay slim. If you are fairly active, you might be able to use as many as 20 calories per pound. Some laborers and athletes use 28 calories per pound of bodyweight each day!

Obviously, it would be difficult to determine exactly how many calories you would need to maintain your ideal weight, which would depend upon how active you are. You'll have to be guided by experience. If you find yourself gaining weight, you'll have to reduce your intake of calories or get more exercise.

If you eat strictly natural foods, it's not likely that you'll exceed your calorie needs if you are fairly active. But if you want to check your calorie intake, figure about 13 calories per pound of bodyweight if you are inactive and about 15 calories per pound of bodyweight if you are fairly active. List all the foods you eat in one day and then check them against a comprehensive list giving the calorie content of all foods. You can find such a list in booklets sold in almost any drug store or newsstand. (You can find the calorie content of many commonly used natural foods listed in Chapter 6.)

Adult Calorie Allowances for Normal Physical Activity

Here is a chart showing the average calorie needs for physically active adults.

Calorie Allowances for Men

Weight	25 years	45 years	65 years
110	2,300	2,050	1,750
120	2,400	2,200	1,850
130	2,550	2,300	1,950
140	2,700	2,450	2,050
150	2,850	2,550	2,150
160	3,000	2,700	2,250
170	3,100	2,800	2,350
180	3,250	2,950	2,450
190	3,400	3,050	2,600

Calorie Allowances for Women

Weight	25 years	45 years	65 years
90	1,600	1,500	1,250
100	1,750	1,600	1,350
110	1,900	1,700	1,450
120	2,000	1,800	1,500
130	2,100	1,900	1,600
140	2,250	2,050	1,700
150	2,350	2,150	1,800
160	2,500	2,250	1,900

The average American adult consumes 3,300 calories a day, but, according to the National Research Council of the National Academy of Sciences, this is far too many. Men 18 to 35 should consume 2,900 calories per day, and women in that age group should get 2,100 calories. Men 35 to 55 should take in no more than 2,600 calories; women, 1,900 calories. Men 55 to 75 years old should consume 2,200 calories per day, and women only 1,600.

Serve Low-Calorie Party Snacks

When you go to a bridge party or social function where snacks or "refreshments" are served, chances are they'll be the refined, high-calorie variety. Potato chips, nuts roasted in oil, processed cheese dip, crackers, and cookies, for example, are popular snack items, and they're loaded with empty calories. After reading this book, you'll know better than to do more than sample such goodies. Your friends, however, may not be able to resist satisfying their taste for such fat-building snacks.

The next time you have an opportunity to serve party snacks in your own home, you can take advantage of your knowledge of nutrition to serve nutritious *natural* snacks. A mixture of raw sunflower seeds, pumpkin seeds, and raisins, for example, is delicious. Seeds and nuts are fairly rich in calories, but they'll satisfy your appetite more readily than a processed snack that contains nothing but calories.

Fresh fruit with cottage cheese makes a delicious snack that is low in calories. Cold melon is refreshing during the summer months. Cubes of yellow cheese with whole wheat crackers are much more delicious than greasy potato chips and processed cheese dip. Natural (unhydrogenated) peanut butter smeared on fruit or whole-grain crackers is a taste treat that children and adults alike can appreciate. You can serve a mixture of unsweetened fruit juices rather than soft drinks, coffee, tea, or alcohol. You can find many natural snack items in a health food store. Many grocery stores now sell ice cream that contains all-natural ingredients. (See Chapter 10 for recipes covering a variety of snack items.)

Persons who are on a low-calorie reducing diet might prefer celery sticks with cottage cheese and vegetable juice. Many vegetables are delicious when cut into sticks and served raw. If you make your own whole-grain bread, why not serve half slices of bread with a little cheese and fruit?

With a little imagination, you can serve *original* snacks that will improve the health of your guests. Although such snacks are likely to be higher in calories than the steamed vegetables and broiled meats you serve for dinner, an occasional high-calorie snack won't contribute to overweight if it is fresh, natural, and wholesome. In fact, such snacks will satisfy your appetite so thoroughly that you'll eat *less* at mealtime, thus consuming fewer calories than you normally would.

Natural food snacks won't artificially stimulate your taste buds. And once you become accustomed to the delicious taste of natural foods, you'll refuse to eat processed foods. The result will be a slimmer, healthier body.

SUMMARY

1. Once your weight has been reduced to a desired level, you might be able to start eating some of your favorite high-calorie natural foods.

2. On a fat-fighting diet in which you are simply trying to maintain your ideal weight, you can be guided by your weight and your physical appearance in evaluating the effects of the foods you eat.

3. The only difference between a fat-disintegrator diet and a fat-fighting diet is that you may be more liberal in your use of natural foods.

4. When you discover during a weekly weighing that you are a couple of pounds over your ideal weight, cut back on high-calorie foods and increase your physical activity.

5. No matter what type of diet you're on or what your weight might be, you should eat some of all the basic natural foods to assure good health.

6. Even if you are no longer overweight, you should continue to avoid the use of sugar and white-flour products.

7. Combining physical activity with a balanced natural-foods diet is the best way to fight fat if you like to eat.

8. Remember that too much animal fat in the diet can harden the arteries of skinny and fat people alike. Too much vegetable oil can speed the aging process and cause cancer.

9. Very active persons need more calories than sedentary persons in order to maintain an ideal weight, but a low-calorie diet that supplies adequate amounts of protein, vitamins, and minerals is more conducive to a long life.

10. When you must serve snacks at a social function, use natural-food snacks rather than processed or packaged snacks.

9

How to Overcome Special Food Problems with Fat-Fighting Foods

No matter what type of ailment you might be suffering from, a balanced natural-foods diet, such as that recommended in the beginning of this book, will usually help combat the problem. An improvement in your general health will help relieve as well as prevent many common ailments. In some cases, however, it might be necessary to make a few special changes in your diet. If you are allergic to milk or wheat, for example, or if you suffer from kidney stones, gout, stomach ulcers, diabetes, soft bones, hardened arteries, diverticulitis, constipation, hemorrhoids, anemia, cystitis, high blood pressure, or kidney disease, you'll find useful guidance in this chapter. With the right diet, *you can relieve symptoms while you reduce your bodyweight.*

You should, of course, always see your doctor when you develop an ailment of any kind. Everything you learn in this chapter pertaining to your particular ailment will fit right in with your doctor's advice. If you have a "tendency" toward some of these ailments, or if you are in an early stage of developing the ailments, you may be able to *prevent* their development with proper dietary procedures.

EXAMPLES OF REDUCING DIETS
USED TO TREAT AILMENTS

Just to give you a few examples of how you can use a reducing diet to relieve the symptoms of disease, consider the cases of Herschel R., Rosa W., and Byron E.

How Herschel R. Solved His Problems with My Reducing Diet

Herschel R. was 50 pounds overweight and suffered from gout and kidney stones when he started my fat-disintegrator diet. He lost the entire 50 pounds in only 16 weeks. After one year of maintaining a normal bodyweight, he had not suffered from another attack of gout or kidney stones! All he had to do to accomplish this was to make a few simple changes in his diet, such as eating less of certain protein-rich foods and more of the type of foods that reduce the amount of acid in the urine. The changes he made in his diet did not in any way diminish the effectiveness of his reducing diet.

How Rosa W. Stopped Chronic Diarrhea by Changing Her Diet

Rosa W. suffered from chronic diarrhea. A description of her stool revealed a probable allergy to gluten, a substance found in wheat, rye, oats, and barley. "I have always heard that wheat products are good for you," she insisted, "so I have started eating whole-wheat bread and cereals every day."

When I persuaded Rosa to give up wheat and substitute corn and soybean products, her symptoms immediately disappeared. She went on to lose 20 pounds of excess fat in one month. Had Rosa continued to eat wheat products, she would have lost an excessive amount of weight from a nutritional deficiency (as a result of the diarrhea) and would have ruined her health.

How Byron E. Relieved Three Ailments with a Reducing Diet

Byron E. was an obese plumber who suffered from constipation, hemorrhoids, and a diaphragmatic hernia. "My doctor put me on a bland diet 15 years ago when I suffered an acute attack of diarrhea caused by diverticulitis," he explained. "Since then, I've gained 75 pounds. I also now suffer from constipation and hemorrhoids."

Byron was still on the bland diet prescribed by his doctor 15 years ago! He still had an occasional bout with diarrhea, but most of the time he suffered from constipation. Straining to empty his bowels caused swelling and bleeding of his hemorrhoids.

I put Byron on my natural foods reducing diet, with plenty of cellulose supplied by fresh fruits and vegetables. It took him several months to lose his excess body fat, but there was immediate improvement in his constipation and his hemorrhoids. So far, he has not had another bout with diarrhea.

All of Byron's problems stemmed from his diet. The same bland diet that was adding weight to his body was clogging his bowels, which in turn aggravated his hemorrhoids and his colon condition. The simple changes made in switching to a diet of natural foods solved his problems.

HOW TO USE A REDUCING DIET TO RELIEVE OR PREVENT HARDENED AND CLOGGED ARTERIES

Each year, about 1.5 million Americans are afflicted with heart attacks and strokes, accounting for 54 percent of all deaths. Nearly 700,000 people die from heart attacks alone! Most of these deaths are the result of hardened and clogged arteries that have been diseased by years of bad eating habits. Cholesterol, triglycerides, and lipoproteins, for example, are forms of hard fat that accumulate in the arteries when there is an excessive amount of animal fat, sugar, and refined carbohydrates in the diet.

The fat-disintegrator diet outlined in this book will automatically reduce blood fat and combat hardened arteries while reducing your bodyweight. Eliminating the sugar and refined carbohydrates in your diet and reducing your intake of animal fat will virtually eliminate the major sources of the type of hard fat that damages arteries. The small amount of vegetable oil you use on your green salads will supply the essential "soft" fatty acids your body needs to dissolve or soften the hard fat that should normally circulate in your arteries.

Even after you have reduced your bodyweight, you can stay on my fat-disintegrator diet for the rest of your life in order to protect your arteries and keep your body lean.

HOW TO CORRECT ANEMIA WHILE ON A REDUCING DIET

According to *Human Nutrition,* published by the U.S. Department of Agriculture, "Nutritional anemia is one of the most widely occurring deficiencies." *Iron deficiency* is the most common cause of nutritional anemia. Deficiencies in folic acid, Vitamin B_{12}, and protein are also often involved.

Iron, Vitamin B_{12}, and protein are best supplied by meats and other animal products. Leafy vegetables are among the best sources of folic acid. Vegetarians who do not include milk, eggs, or cheese in their diet may develop anemia from a Vitamin B_{12} deficiency. Persons who eat meats but no vegetables may be deficient in folic acid, and so on.

Obviously, every reducing diet must contain both vegetables and animal products in order to keep the blood healthy. This is one reason why I do not recommend reducing diets that exclude some of the basic natural foods.

My fat-disintegrator and fat-fighting diets supply balanced amounts of *all* the vitamins and minerals you need to build rich, red blood. If you are anemic, however, your physician may prescribe Vitamin B_{12} or an iron supplement to rebuild your blood as rapidly as possible. When the red blood cells are deficient in iron, you can safely assume that all the organs of your body are also deficient in iron. Considering the small amount of iron that can be absorbed each day from the foods of a reducing diet, you may have to have some additional iron to rebuild your health. Without an iron supplement, it would take a long time to correct a nutritional anemia, and until the iron levels of your tissues and organs are restored to normal, an iron deficiency in your blood would persist. Some persons may need hydrochloric acid tablets and other supplements to aid the absorption of iron. Let your doctor decide what is causing your anemia and then follow his advice. In the meantime, supplement your diet with desiccated liver tablets for a natural source of iron. Eat fresh, cooked liver as often as possible.

Prevention is the best treatment for nutritional anemia. So be sure to follow my balanced reducing diet rather than one of the fad diets that reduce you "overnight."

COMBAT CONSTIPATION WITH BRAN AND CELLULOSE

Constipation is so common in the United States that it's often called the "great American disease." The primary reason for so much constipation is that most Americans eat excessive amounts of refined and processed foods (the same foods that cause overweight!). Without bran and cellulose in the diet, there is not sufficient stimulation for the bowels. As a result, sticky food residue simply accumulates in the colon where it becomes packed and hardened.

Reducing diets that stress meats, fats, milk, and other low-residue, high-protein foods commonly result in constipation. Without fruits, vegetables, cereals, and other foods that contain indigestible fiber, cellulose, or bran, constipation is inevitable.

The same dietary deficiencies that cause constipation can also cause colon cancer, diverticulitis, hemorrhoids, and other common bowel diseases. So be sure to avoid those zero carbohydrate diets that exclude fruits, cereals, and vegetables.

There is now some evidence to indicate that too much beef in the diet, like too much refined carbohydrate, may be a cause of colon cancer (especially if the beef contains hormones). It's much better to lose weight a little slower on a balanced diet of natural foods than to shed weight rapidly on a specialized fad diet, such as a meat diet.

If you follow my natural foods reducing diet, it's not likely that you'll ever suffer from constipation. If you do, adding a couple tablespoons of bran to your meals or simply "fasting" on raw fruits and vegetables for a couple of days will wake up your bowels. A large amount of cellulose in your intestinal tract will hold moisture as well as stimulate bowel movements. Be sure to drink plenty of water and keep regular toilet appointments. You can get pure, unprocessed bran in any health food store.

Note: Failure to have a bowel movement for a couple of days does not necessarily mean that you are constipated. If you do miss two or three days, however, and your stool is hard or in the shape of marbles, an enema may be helpful in breaking up impactions in your colon.

Warning: While a small amount of bran in the diet helps prevent constipation, an excessive amount of bran might accumulate in diverticula or pouches and become impacted. Put a little bran in your cereals, in bread, meat loaf, and other foods prepared at home, and then get as much cellulose as you can from fresh fruits and vegetables. I personally feel that cellulose is more beneficial than bran·for good bowel health.

PROCEED CAUTIOUSLY WITH DIVERTICULITIS

When there is not sufficient fiber or cellulose in the diet, the sticky, constipating residue that accumulates in the lower bowel creates pressure that produces small balloons or pouches in the colon walls. When these pouches become clogged or inflamed, there may be pain, spasm, constipation, or diarrhea.

If you already have diverticulitis (which must be diagnosed by an X-ray examination), you may have to reduce your intake of foods that contain bran, seeds, husks, nuts, and other forms of roughage that might accumulate in inflamed pouches. It might be necessary to cook your fruits and vegetables so that they won't be coarse enough to trigger diarrhea or intestinal spasms.

Your reducing diet won't be affected by temporarily eliminating raw foods, but you should gradually begin eating fresh fruits and raw salads whenever symptoms subside. You *must* have fiber or cellulose in your intestinal tract to "sweep out" the pouches and aid bowel movements. A prolonged diet of "soft" foods may only clog the pouches and result in recurring attacks of diverticulitis.

Persons who are fortunate enough to begin a diet of natural foods *before* bowel troubles develop can usually *prevent* them.

HOW TO HEAL ULCERS BY EATING NATURALLY ON A REDUCING DIET

Peptic ulcer is the most common disease of the digestive tract. Doctors used to believe that a special bland or soft diet, such as milk and crackers, was essential in the healing of a stomach ulcer. The consensus now, however, is that a variety of natural foods may be just as effective. The trick is to keep something in your stomach to absorb the excess acid. Between-meal snacks of cottage cheese, lean meat, broiled chicken, or fish, for example, are often recommended.

Many people with an ulcer can eat normally if they eat frequently, chew their foods thoroughly, and avoid alcohol, coffee, and spicy foods. Eating natural foods between meals, as I suggested in my fat-disintegrator and fat-fighting diets, will help heal your ulcer as well as reduce your bodyweight.

Note: If your ulcer begins to bleed, your stools will be black and tarry. Cut back on your raw fruits and vegetables and see your doctor. *You should always seek medical attention when you have stomach pain of any kind.*

HOW TO FIGHT GOUT WITH FOOD

Gout is a common complication of reducing diets that result in a rapid weight loss. A large amount of uric acid released by the breakdown of fat and muscle tissue accumulates in the joints to cause severe pain and swelling. Some high-protein diets trigger the development of gout in susceptible persons by supplying uric acid when animal organs, meats, fish, and poultry are being digested. Fasting may also result in an increase in the amount of uric acid in the blood.

If your body is normal and healthy, your kidneys will be able to eliminate the uric acid that might otherwise accumulate in your body. Once you develop gout, however, you must forever be careful to avoid eating excessive amounts of protein foods that contain purine or uric acid. Weight loss must be limited to a couple of pounds a week, and fasting must be avoided.

If you have never had gout before, it's not likely that you ever will on my fat-disintegrator or fat-fighting diet. If you are already suffering from gout, you must go easy on meat, fish, and poultry and try to get most of your protein from skim milk, eggs, and cottage cheese. Nuts and seeds also contain protein, but they are high in fat. Gelatin is a pure protein, but since it is not a *complete* protein, it can be used only in conjunction with other foods containing protein.

Whole wheat contains purine, so you may have to substitute corn bread for whole wheat bread. Whole-grain cereals can be replaced with smaller amounts of grits or cream of wheat.

Fresh fruits, vegetables, and juices will help prevent the formation of uric acid stones by alkalizing your urine. When you are actually suffering from gout, you should *drink up to three quarts of liquids daily* to flush the uric acid out of your body. Vegetable juices and plenty of water should to the trick.

Note: If your big toe, wrist, or some other joint swells and throbs with pain, see your doctor. A simple blood test will reveal whether you have gout or not. If you do not have gout, you should continue to include generous amounts of fish and poultry in your reducing diet.

In severe cases of gout, the body may be *manufacturing* excessive amounts of uric acid. Whenever this is the case, a physician may have to prescribe special medication to keep the gout under control.

HOW TO STRENGTHEN SOFT BONES
WITH DIETARY PROCEDURES

The importance of a balanced diet, especially when it is a reducing diet, is often dramatically revealed in the bones of persons suffering from a calcium deficiency. Loose teeth and soft vertebrae, for example, are disgracefully common. Approximately 30 percent of all women and 20 percent of all men over the age of 50 have vertebrae that are soft enough to permit the development of compression and deformity. Doctors call this disease osteoporosis.

The calcium-rich milk products recommended in my reducing diet will help prevent the development of osteoporosis, but only if you follow a balanced diet. Many other elements, such as phosphorus, Vitamin D, fluoride, and magnesium, are also important in the formation of bone. If a diet is unbalanced, a deficiency (or an excess) of any one of the vitamins and minerals needed to build bone may result in soft bones. Some of the high-protein "water diets," in which only meats and water are allowed, are deficient in calcium. An excessive amount of phosphorus supplied by a "protein diet" can *create* a calcium deficiency by causing calcium to be excreted from the body.

A balanced reducing diet, such as that outlined in this book, maintains a balance of calcium, phosphorus, and other food elements needed to build and maintain good health.

If you develop soft bones in spite of a good diet that includes milk products, you might be deficient in the stomach acid you need to absorb calcium. Or you might be having trouble with your parathyroid gland. Some women who have gone through the menopause or have had their ovaries removed must take estrogen to prevent loss of calcium from their bones.

Stomach acid deficiency is a common cause of bone softening in older people. Whenever this is present, the addition of hydrochloric acid tablets to a balanced diet might solve the problem. Bone meal tablets may be added to meals for additional calcium. You need at least 800 milligrams of calcium a day to maintain normal bones. If your bones are soft, you may need up to 1,500 milligrams of calcium each day to construct new bone.

Note: Persons who are totally inactive will lose calcium from their bones regardless of how well-balanced their meals may be. So there are good reasons why you should remain physically active, even if diet alone seems to reduce your bodyweight.

HOW TO ALTER YOUR DIET TO COMBAT KIDNEY STONES

If your body functions normally, it's not likely that you'll ever develop a kidney stone on a balanced diet of natural foods. Stones can develop, however, when there is a deficiency in certain nutrients, notably pyridoxine (Vitamine B_6) and magnesium. An excessive amount of Vitamin D in the diet can also be a factor, and so can inactivity or a hyperactive parathyroid gland. For the most part, however, very little is known about the cause of kidney stones.

Acidify Your Urine to Prevent Calcium Phosphate Stones

Once a stone does form, the type of stone you have will determine what changes you must make in your diet. If your doctor tells you that you have a *calcium phosphate stone,* you'll have to eat more of the foods that increase the amount of *acid* in your urine, since phosphate stones form more readily in alkaline urine.

Meat, eggs, fowl, fish, and whole-grain products leave an acid residue. *Plums and cranberries* are the only fresh fruits I know of that contribute acid to the urine.

You'll have to avoid the use of antacids and alkalies, especially in combination with milk. The use of milk should be limited. Milk enriched with Vitamin D should be completely avoided.

Aluminum hydroxide gel, prescribed by your doctor, will combine with excess dietary phosphorus so that it can be eliminated by your bowels. The calcium in your urine can then be eliminated without forming stones. You should, of course, drink plenty of water.

Obviously, a diet that's low in calcium and phosphorus must be supervised by a physician in order to avoid a mineral deficiency that might weaken your bones.

Alkalize Your Urine to Prevent Calcium Oxalate Stones

Oxalate stones form in an acid urine. This means that if you have *calcium oxalate stones,* you'll have to eat foods that *alkalize* your urine.

Liberal use of fruits and vegetables and their juices will alkalize your urine and help prevent the formation of stones. Meat, fowl, cheese, eggs, fish, and cereals will have to be restricted, and milk limited to about one pint per day.

Oral supplements of magnesium and Vitamin B_6, with about two quarts of water a day, have proven to be useful in preventing the formation of oxalate stones.

A NATURAL FOODS REDUCING DIET IS A GOOD DIET FOR DIABETES

An excessive amount of sugar and refined carbohydrate in the diet, in addition to causing overweight, can cause diabetes by overworking the pancreas. Most diabetics inherit a tendency to develop the disease, but it can often be prevented or controlled with the proper diet. Because of the bad eating habits of most Americans, about one in 20 has diabetes or is potentially diabetic, with the diabetic population increasing each year.

If you follow my natural-foods reducing diet and eliminate sugar and refined carbohydrates from your diet as I suggested, your chances of developing diabetes are reduced almost to zero. If you are already diabetic, a diet limited to lean meats, fish, poultry, eggs, fresh fruits, vegetables, raw salads, skim milk, whole-grain products, and other natural foods may allow you to control the disease without taking insulin. You may even be able to eat generous quantities of fresh fruit without raising your blood sugar. *The same natural-foods diet that I recommend for reducing your bodyweight is the best diet for controlling diabetes.*

An occasional blood sugar test by your family physician will reveal whether you need insulin or not. If you do take insulin, a diet of natural foods, properly balanced, may reduce your need for injections of insulin. This must be determined by a physician, however, on the basis of repeated blood tests.

The mineral chromium has been used successfully in preventing the development of diabetes. Wheat germ, bran, and other foods rich in fiber are good sources of chromium. Sugar in the diet tends to result in a chromium deficiency. In addition to contributing an excessive amount of sugar to the blood, refined carbohydrates have been stripped of all their fiber.

Note: With the average American eating about 120 pounds of sugar each year, along with great quantities of refined carbohydrates, it's no wonder that so many people have diabetes. You should not eat any sugar at all if you can avoid it. Your body gets all the sugar it needs from the natural carbohydrates in your diet.

Even a diabetic must have a certain amount of natural carbohydrate. If the diet is properly balanced with natural foods, the body will not convert an excessive amount of the carbohydrate to sugar.

IF YOU ARE ALLERGIC TO WHEAT . . .

About one person in every 1,000 is allergic to gluten, a type of protein found in wheat, rye, oats, and barley. The result is celiac disease or diarrhea, which is characterized by foamy, light-colored stools that contain a considerable amount of fat and calcium soap. Poor absorption of fat-soluble vitamins (A, D, E, and K) and other nutrients as a result of the diarrhea leads to the development of anemia, skin disease, soft bones, loose teeth, and other symptoms.

The only treatment for celiac disease is to *avoid all cereal grains except corn and rice.* Since beer and ale often contain grain residue, they, too, must be avoided. Of course, on a fat-disintegrator or fat-fighting diet, you don't need beer or ale anyway.

If you must use flour in the preparation of bread or rolls, you can use flour made from corn, rice, soybeans, and potatoes. Remember, however, that any flour product is fairly high in calories and must be used sparingly.

Note: Many processed foods contain refined wheat flour. If you eat completely natural foods, you'll be able to avoid hidden wheat in packaged foods.

Warning: Some reducing diets recommend the use of gluten bread, since it is high in protein and low in carbohydrate. If you use such bread, watch for any signs of gluten allergy, namely diarrhea.

HOW TO RELIEVE CYSTITIS WITH DIETARY MEASURES

The urine is normally slightly acid. When the bladder and urethra are raw and inflamed, however, the acid urine can cause burning pain that further erodes raw tissues. Most cystitis is the result of infection rather than dietary indiscretion.

When everything is normal, acid urine helps *combat* infection. But once the bladder and the urethra have become raw and inflamed, it may be necessary to alter your diet a little in order to *alkalize* your urine. This will help relieve the irritation until healing occurs. Drink a glass of water or fruit juice every half hour. The more liquids you drink the better, since this will flush out your bladder and dilute your urine so that it will be less irritating. It's the juice that alkalizes your urine, so drink as much juice as possible.

In severe cases, a little baking soda in water or lemonade can be used. A low-protein diet consisting mainly of fresh fruits and vegetables, with very little meat, bread, milk, or cereal, will help maintain an alkaline urine.

Vitamin C and cranberry juice are often used to *prevent* urinary infection, since they prevent the growth of bacteria by increasing the amount of acid in the urine. Early infection might be curbed by drinking cranberry juice, but an acid urine might aggravate the raw tissues of an advanced infection.

See your doctor when any type of urinary problem develops. Uncontrolled infections could become serious. If the urine must be made alkaline to relieve burning pain, it might be necessary for your doctor to prescribe an antibiotic to kill the infection.

RELIEVE THE SYMPTOMS OF A DIAPHRAGMATIC HERNIA WITH WEIGHT REDUCTION

When a diaphragmatic or hiatal hernia occurs, a portion of the stomach protrudes up into the chest through an opening in the diaphragm. This may result in chest and abdominal pain after you eat, especially when you are lying down.

If you have a diaphragmatic hernia and you are overweight, chances are you'll experience dramatic relief when your bodyweight has been reduced. So be sure to stick with your diet! If you eat small meals, you probably won't have any trouble with a diaphragmatic hernia. But if you should occasionally lose control of your taste buds and overeat, you may be able to avoid pain, spasm, heartburn, and other symptoms by not lying down after eating. This will keep food from being trapped in the portion of the stomach above the diaphragm.

A diaphragmatic hernia must, of course, be diagnosed by a physician, who can rule out stomach ulcers and heart trouble. Call your doctor for a checkup when you experience any kind of chest or abdominal pain.

HEMORRHOIDS CAN BE CAUSED BY A BAD DIET

The same kind of diet that causes overweight, diverticulitis, and colon cancer can also cause hemorrhoids! Straining to empty a bowel that is clogged with the sticky residue of refined and processed foods causes the rectal and anal veins to swell with blood, resulting in varicose veins. When one of these veins ruptures, there may be a considerable amount of bleeding.

If you don't already have itching, burning hemorrhoids, a natural foods diet that is rich in bran and cellulose will help *prevent* them. If you already have a bad case of hemorrhoids, you may have to reduce the amount of bran and raw cellulose in your diet in order to relieve painful irritation of inflamed and swollen veins. It's very important, however, to keep enough roughage in your diet to prevent constipation. Otherwise, straining to empty your bowels will make your hemorrhoids worse.

If you must temporarily reduce the amount of roughage in your diet until your hemorrhoids are no longer inflamed, be sure to include a natural bulk laxative, such as psyllium seed extract, to make sure that you do not become constipated. Cooked vegetables will help maintain normal bowel movements. When symptoms subside, begin including larger amounts of whole-grain products, raw fruits and vegetables, and other foods rich in bran and cellulose.

CONTROLLING THE SODIUM IN YOUR DIET

For best results on a reducing diet, you should not eat salted foods or use table salt. Too much salt in your diet can force your body to retain an excessive amount of water. It can also harden your arteries and raise your blood pressure. You can get all the salt you need from natural foods.

The average person consumes from two to three teaspoons of salt each day, which is equivalent to 3,000 to 6,000 milligrams of sodium. If you avoid salty foods and do not use table salt, your diet will supply about 2,000 to 3,000 milligrams of sodium. If your doctor puts you on a special low-sodium diet that excludes *foods* that are naturally rich in sodium, your sodium intake will be reduced to less than 1,000 milligrams.

Remember that it's the *sodium* in salt that does the damage. Refined and processed foods are often loaded with sodium. If you follow my fat-disintegrator diet, you'll be using a minimum amount of salt, and you won't be eating any refined and processed foods at all.

If you have high blood pressure, hardened arteries, or "water in your tissues," your doctor might ask you to eliminate table salt completely. If he does, you can use a vegetable salt that does not contain sodium chloride. Be sure to read the labels on any canned or packaged foods you might eat. If they contain sodium in any form, including artificial sweeteners or preservatives, do not eat them. If you must use baking powder, use a sodium-free variety.

The drinking water in some areas of the country is high in sodium. Check with your local water department or have a sample of your water analyzed. Water softeners increase the sodium content of water greatly. If you find it necessary to drink distilled or bottled water in order to avoid sodium, it might be a good idea to take a mineral supplement.

The use of an excessive amount of table salt is simply a habit in most cases. If you feel that you have an abnormal craving for salt, have your doctor check the function of your adrenal glands. People with Addison's disease, for example, often retain water and crave salt.

Note: If you do not use table salt, be sure to eat seafood at least once a week to replace the iodine normally supplied by iodized salt. Vegetables sometimes contain iodine, but since the soil is often deficient in iodine, the average person must depend upon seafood or iodized salt for iodine.

A SPECIAL DIET FOR KIDNEY TROUBLE

If you have kidney trouble, your physician may have to prescribe a special diet for you. In some cases, it may be necessary to *reduce* the amount of protein in your diet in order to reduce the workload on your kidneys. Or it may be necessary to *increase* the amount of protein in your diet to compensate for the urinary loss of protein. The type of kidney trouble you have and the stage of its development will determine how much protein your diet must contain. This must be determined by a physician. If your kidneys do not function normally, check with your doctor before altering your diet beyond what is considered a balanced diet.

Since the kidneys normally eliminate the by-products of protein metabolism, an unbalanced high-protein diet, as in an all-meat diet, might overwork healthy kidneys. So for your health's sake, don't be tempted to follow a high-protein "crash diet." If you have a kidney disease that you are not aware of, a "high-protein diet" could result in kidney failure.

HOW TO HANDLE MILK SUGAR ALLERGY

You already know from reading Chapter 2 that many adults do not have the digestive enzyme they need to digest and absorb lactose or milk sugar. The result is diarrhea that flushes essential nutrients from the intestinal tract before they can be absorbed.

If milk disturbs your intestinal tract, avoid milk and get your calcium from *fermented* milk products, such as yogurt or cottage cheese. See Chapter 11 for a soy milk recipe. Soy milk is rich in protein and can be enriched with calcium by adding calcium lactate.

SUMMARY

1. A natural-foods reducing diet helps *prevent* the development of many common ailments.

2. No matter what type of ailment you might be suffering from, there are special diets that you can follow to relieve symptoms while you reduce your bodyweight.

3. Many common ailments, such as arteriosclerosis, constipation, diverticulitis, stomach ulcers, osteoporosis, diabetes, and hemorrhoids, can be relieved with the same simple diet that I recommend for reducing body fat.

4. A natural foods diet prevents the development of anemia, but if you are already anemic you should take an iron or Vitamin B_{12} supplement prescribed by your family physician.

5. Frequent small meals of natural foods will often help heal a stomach ulcer by absorbing excess stomach acid.

6. If you suffer from gout, you may have to depend more upon eggs, cheese, and skimmed milk (or fermented milk products) for your protein and eat less meat, fish, and poultry.

7. If you develop soft bones or loose teeth in spite of a good diet, you may need to add hydrochloric acid tablets to your meals to aid absorption of calcium.

8. The type of kidney stone you have will determine whether you should eat foods that leave an acid or an alkaline residue.

9. Persons allergic to the gluten in wheat will have to avoid wheat, rye, oats, barley, and their products.

10. If you have kidney disease, the amount of protein in your diet should be prescribed by a physician.

10

Recipes for Fighting Fat

The best way to prepare natural foods is to use *simple cooking methods* that do not require special ingredients. When you cook cabbage, for example, all you have to do is steam the cabbage a little, add a small amount of salt, and then enjoy the *true taste* of cabbage. Any fresh, natural food that cannot be eaten raw should be cooked as little as possible to preserve nutrients as well as taste. Properly prepared, natural foods are delicious.

If you use the cooking methods I recommended in Chapter 4, you really do not need a recipe book to guide you in preparing the basic natural foods. Any food made more appetizing by "gourmet cooking" or by special seasoning tends to increase your intake of calories by stimulating your appetite. Added ingredients usually also mean added calories.

There are, however, ways to prepare natural foods to *increase* their nutritional value so that you can eat less, safely. Adding bran and bone meal to meat loaf or to home-cooked bread, for example, adds nutrients without adding calories. The use of herbs, spices, and bouillon in cooking can improve the taste of essential vegetables that you may not normally enjoy eating. Combining certain foods will give you the variety you need to keep eating interesting.

In this chapter, you'll learn how to prepare and combine certain natural foods in special ways for better taste as well as for better health. None of the recipes call for white sugar, flour, corn starch, and other refined ingredients. *All* of the recipes build health without building up body fat.

Remember that a recipe is only a guide. You can change any recipe—or you can write your own to suit your taste.

HEALTH FOODS ARE FOR EVERYONE!

If you have reservations about eating "health foods," remember that true health foods are simply fresh, natural foods that build good health. *The trend is back to eating natural foods,* regardless of your bodyweight. Doctors are advising people to avoid the refined and processed foods that tear down health and build up body fat. You can go on a natural foods diet and reduce your bodyweight without any obvious indication that you are on a reducing diet. You'll simply be in step with the times.

Just about everyone is now aware of the dangers of artificial additives in processed foods. So don't be afraid to publicly express your preference for fresh, natural foods. Be proud that you know the difference. You're in good company with millions of intelligent people who have the good sense and the courage to eat what is best for their health.

No matter how you feel about eating for health, *you should eat natural foods if you want to eat generously and lose weight.* If you want to make your diet more interesting, use a natural foods cookbook to put a little variety in your cooking. You'll find a few health-food recipes in this chapter, all using the type of foods I recommend in my fat-disintegrator diet. Remember, however, to use the simple cooking methods described in Chapter 4 to prepare the major portion of your diet. You may then occasionally use some of the recipes in this chapter for adventures in eating and to test your culinary skills.

EAT YOUR WAY TO A NEW WAY OF LIFE

Once you have become accustomed to preparing natural foods, you'll delight in treating your family and your friends with natural-foods dishes. You'll thrive on the taste and the effects of dishes fortified with wheat germ, bone meal, brewer's yeast, powdered skimmed milk, and other concentrated food products that add taste as well as nutrients. You'll have more pep and vitality. And as the pounds melt away, you'll enjoy a new way of life.

Visit your local book store and look for books that supply information on the selection and preparation of natural foods. Eat and enjoy with a clear conscience! With natural foods, you'll reap the benefits of better health, a longer life, and a slimmer body.

Special note: All temperatures given in the preparation of foods and recipes are based on a Fahrenheit scale.

TIPS ON HOW TO COOK MEATS AND POULTRY

On a fat-disintegrator or fat-fighting diet, meats and poultry should always be cooked to *reduce* the amount of fat they contain. This usually means trimming away the visible fat *before* cooking and then roasting, broiling, or barbecuing the meat so that cooked-out fat can be drained away. Frying should be avoided whenever possible.

Just to make sure that you cook your meats properly, review these cooking tips before you consider some of the more unusual recipes.

How to Roast Meat

Meat cooked slowly at a lower temperature is juicier and more tender than meat cooked rapidly at a high temperature. *Oven roasting* is the best way to cook meat slowly.

Trim away all surface fat except for a thin layer. Place the meat on a low rack in a shallow pan, fat side up so that the meat will be self-basting. Heat the oven to 325 degrees. Roast the meat to a desired degree of doneness.

If you use a meat thermometer to roast beef, insert the thermometer into the center of the thickest portion of the meat (so that the thermometer won't touch the bone). The temperature of the center of the meat will accurately reflect the degree of doneness. When the temperature reaches 170 degrees Fahrenheit, for example, the meat is well done; 160 degrees is medium, and 140 degrees is rare. Generally, it takes about 45 minutes per pound to cook beef well done. Pork should always be cooked until it is well done in order to kill parasites. You should *never* eat pork that has a pink color.

Poultry can be roasted in the same manner as beef and other meats—in an oven at 325 degrees in a shallow *uncovered* pan.

Broiling for Quick Cooking

When you want to cook smaller pieces of meat more rapidly, you place the meat on a broiler pan so that the top of the meat will be three to six inches from the source of the heat, depending upon how brown you want the meat and whether your oven is gas or electric. When one side has browned, sprinkle the browned surface with salt and then turn it over and brown the other side.

Note: It's best *not* to preheat the oven when you broil meat, and you should leave the oven door *open*.

Outdoor Barbecuing

Barbecuing allows you to brown meats without overcooking them. And it gives you an opportunity to entertain yourself and your family with outdoor cooking. Special barbecue sauces can be used to flavor the meat or poultry in a delicious and spectacular manner.

When the charcoal has been ignited and is ready for cooking, place the meat on the grill so that it will be three or more inches above the coals. Place the fat side of the meat *down* during the first half of the cooking. Lean meat or poultry can be brushed with vegetable oil when it is first placed on the rack and again when it is turned over. You should not have to turn the meat more than once. You may, of course, use a meat thermometer to determine when a thick piece of meat is adequately cooked.

Note: Do not apply barbecue sauce until the meat is nearly done—about 15 minutes before serving.

Barbecued Beef or Chicken on a Skewer

½ cup vinegar
1 garlic clove, chopped
1 tablespoon chopped chili pepper
1 teaspoon powdered cumin
½ teaspoon salt
black pepper
8 ounces steak or chicken cut into bite-size pieces
1 medium green pepper, cut into sections
½ cup large mushrooms
1 cup cherry tomatoes

Combine all ingredients except tomatoes, green pepper, mushrooms, and the beef or chicken to make a marinade. Marinate the beef or poultry for two hours and then place it on the skewer alternately with the green pepper, tomatoes, and mushrooms. Cook over coals until brown. Makes one dinner serving.

Note: Use your imagination. Use onions, lemon slices, or anything you like on a skewer.

Tomato Barbecue Sauce

If you prefer tomato sauce on your barbecue, try this recipe.

1 can (46 fluid ounces) tomato juice
3 tablespoons vinegar
2 tablespoons dehydrated onion flakes
2 tablespoons mustard
1 tablespoon lemon juice
1 tablespoon Worcestershire sauce
½ teaspoon garlic powder
½ teaspoon barbecue spice
3 tablespoons brown sugar or honey

Combine all ingredients in a saucepan and heat until mixture thickens.

Chicken Hash

Chicken is best baked, broiled, or barbecued. But when you have leftover chicken, you can make a delicious chicken hash.

12 ounces of diced chicken, without bones or skin
2 medium potatoes, boiled and diced
1 medium chopped green pepper
½ cup cooked, diced celery
2 tablespoons diced pimento
1 teaspoon dehydrated onion flakes
1 cup chicken bouillon
½ cup tomato juice, divided into 2 servings
2 medium tomatoes, sliced

Combine chicken, potatoes, pepper, celery, and pimento and chop fine. Divide into two dishes and add onion flakes, bouillon, and tomato juice to each dish. Top with tomato slices and bake at 350 degrees for 30 minutes. Makes two dinner servings.

Broiled Veal Chops

Since veal is lower in fat than most meats, it is a good meat for any reducing diet. Sprinkle tenderloin or veal chops with salt and broil until brown on both sides. Garlic and tomatoes, with mushrooms, marjoram, or rosemary, enhance the taste of veal.

Baked Veal and Vegetable Casserole

Remember that it's better to prepare meats in a simple manner than to cook them in a casserole. A casserole can be used occasionally, however, for a one-dish meal.

1½ pounds veal, sliced thin and cut into 2-inch squares
2 cups chicken bouillon
4 ounces yellow turnip, diced
4 ounces onion, diced
4 ounces carrot, diced
½ cup mushrooms
1 teaspoon minced parsley
1 garlic clove, mashed
dash of marjoram

Cover veal with bouillon in a saucepan and poach gently until veal shows no trace of pink color. Drain veal and place in casserole. Mix in other ingredients, cover, and bake at 325 degrees for one hour.

Healthy Meat Loaf

2 slices of whole-wheat bread crumbled into ½ cup skim milk

1 egg

1 or 2 shredded onions

1 minced garlic clove

¼ cup wheat germ

1½ pounds lean ground beef

½ pound pork sausage

1½ teaspoons salt

2 tablespoons chopped parsley

¼ teaspoon black pepper

Mix all ingredients and mold into a loaf in a shallow baking dish or pack into a greased loaf pan. Bake at 350 degrees for about one hour—or until meat thermometer registers 185 degrees.

Health-Food Meat Loaf

If you want to work some of your nutritional supplements into your meat loaf, try this recipe for *super health.*

2 eggs

½ teaspoon salt

1 teaspoon bone meal

2 tablespoons brewer's yeast

1 cup sunflower seed meal

½ cup chopped onion

¼ teaspoon black pepper

½ teaspoon sage

1 teaspoon kelp

½ cup shredded carrots

1 pound ground beef

2 parsnips, thinly sliced

2 hard-boiled eggs

Preheat the oven to 300 degrees. Mix the uncooked eggs, salt, bone meal, yeast, sunflower seed meal, onion, pepper, sage, and kelp in a blender. Mix the carrots and beef in a bowl and then mix in the blended mixture. Place a layer of parsnip slices in the bottom of a buttered loaf pan. Put in half of the meat mixture, press the two hard-boiled eggs into the meat, and then put in the remaining meat mixture. Bake one hour or until done. Yields about six servings.

Turkey or Chicken Chow Mein

½ cup (2 ounces) cooked chicken or turkey, cut into cubes
½ medium onion, chopped
2 scallions with 3 inches green top, chopped
½ cup sliced mushrooms
½ cup sliced celery
1 cup chicken stock
1 tablespoon soy sauce
½ cup sprouts
1 tablespoon slivered almonds
2 tablespoons cooked brown rice

Simmer onion, scallions, mushrooms, and celery in chicken stock for five minutes. Stir in soy sauce. Cook for four minutes. Add chicken, sprouts, almonds, and cooked rice and cook for one minute more.

Ground Beef Patties

2 slices whole-wheat bread
1 medium onion
½ cup skimmed milk
2 tightly packed cups of ground lean beef
1 teaspoon salt
black pepper
⅓ cup wheat germ
pinch of sage, basil, or savory

Crumble bread, grate onion, and mix into skim milk. Mix with remaining ingredients. Mold mixture into patties one inch thick and roll in wheat germ or whole-wheat bread crumbs. Bake, broil, or fry.

Stuffed Peppers

4 large red bell peppers
1 pound lean ground beef
1 cup cooked brown rice
1 teaspoon salt
black pepper
⅛ teaspoon each of savory, basil, and marjoram

Cut peppers lengthwise and remove seeds. Place peppers on a rack above boiling water and steam for 10 or 15 minutes or until tender. Mix other ingredients, stuff into peppers, and set in baking pan. Sprinkle with wheat germ and bake in oven at 350 degrees for 20 minutes.

Liver and Onions

1 tablespoon vegetable oil
4 large chopped onions
1 pound of liver, cut into ¾-inch cubes
2 tablespoons sherry or port wine
1 tablespoon salt

Saute the chopped onions in the vegetable oil for five minutes. Then add other ingredients and cook two to four minutes.

Three More Ways to Prepare Liver

Have your butcher cut liver into slices ⅓ of an inch thick. Cut away all the blood vessels and membranes before cooking. If you like, you can marinate liver with chicken bouillon (for at least 30 minutes) to alter its taste.

You can *panbroil* liver in a non-stick skillet for four or five minutes or until it is done on both sides. When the liver is brown, add diced vegetables, such as green pepper, onions, and celery, and simmer in a little boiling water until the vegetables are tender. Salt and pepper to taste.

To *broil* liver, place the liver three or four inches from the source of the heat and cook about two minutes. Sprinkle with lemon juice and minced water cress before serving.

Liver can be *baked* at 350 degrees Fahrenheit until it is tender or for 40 or 50 minutes. Make a complete meal with liver by serving it with two or three steamed vegetables.

Leftover Liver Scramble

If you do not particularly like the taste of liver, and you have some leftover, you can disguise its taste with a tasty egg-and-vegetable scramble.

2 ounces cooked, diced liver
½ medium tomato, diced
½ medium green pepper, chopped
1 tablespoon tomato juice
¼ teaspoon dehydrated onion flakes
salt and pepper
dash of cayenne pepper
1 egg, beaten

Combine tomato, green pepper, tomato juice, onion flakes, salt and pepper and simmer in a skillet until liquid has evaporated and pepper is soft. Add diced liver and stir in egg, scrambling to taste. Makes one luncheon serving.

MEAT SUBSTITUTES

Since soybeans contain a complete protein that is nearly equal to meat, they are often used as a meat substitute.

How to Cook Dried Soybeans

2 cups (1 pound) dried soybeans
cold water
salt to taste

Place the dried beans in a bowl of cold water and let them soak overnight. Remember that the dried beans will increase in size when they absorb water. So be sure to use a large bowl and cover the beans with two or three inches of water.

Place the soaking water and the beans in a heavy kettle. If necessary, add enough extra water to cover the beans. Add a little salt, bring the water to a boil, and then simmer over low heat for three or four hours until the beans are tender.

Flavored Soybeans

If you do not enjoy the taste of soybeans, here's a "flavored" recipe that you might like.

1½ cups dry soybeans
1 cup hot soup stock
½ teaspoon black pepper
2 teaspoons salt
2 tablespoons vegetable oil
1 or 2 minced garlic cloves
1 chopped onion
½ to 1 cup tomato puree
1 tablespoon Worcestershire sauce
1 bay leaf
2 or 4 tablespoons chopped parsley

Soak the soybeans overnight in cold water. Then simmer in soaking water (in a covered pot) for four or five hours until the beans are nearly tender. If additional cooking water is needed, add hot soup stock. When beans are nearly done, add remaining ingredients except chopped parsley and continue cooking in a covered pot until the beans are tender. Then add the chopped parsley.

Soybean Casserole

3 tablespoons vegetable oil
1 cup chopped celery
1 cup chopped onions
2½ cups chopped fresh tomatoes
2 garlic cloves, finely chopped
½ teaspoon salt
½ cup wheat germ
½ cup chicken broth or bouillon
3 tablespoons brewer's yeast
3 tablespoons soy flour
3 cups cooked soybeans

Preheat the oven to 350 degrees. Heat the vegetable oil in a skillet and saute the celery and onions until they are tender.

Then mix all ingredients together and put them into an oiled casserole. Bake 30 minutes. Yields six servings.

Soybean Patties

1 16-ounce can of soybeans or 2 cups cooked soybeans
½ cup wheat germ
1 small onion, finely chopped
½ green pepper, finely chopped
2 eggs, lightly beaten
1 tablespoon soy sauce
1 fresh tomato, pureed in blender
2 tablespoons parsley flakes
1 tablespoon powdered vegetable broth
salt and pepper to taste

Preheat oven to 350 degrees. Drain soybeans and mash with potato masher. Add remaining ingredients and mix thoroughly. Mold into patties and place on a baking sheet. Bake for 25 minutes, turn with spatula, and then bake 15 minutes more. Serves about eight.

FISH RECIPES

Since fish is an excellent low-fat food for a reducing diet, you should eat it as often as possible. Broiling is the easiest and the best way to cook fish.

How to Broil Fish

For best results in broiling, fish should not be more than 1½ inches thick. Brush the fish with vegetable oil to seal in its juices. (Do not add salt until fish is done.)

Place the broiler pan so that it will be about five inches from electric heating unit. Turn the fish after eight to 10 minutes, or when fish turns white. It takes about 15 minutes to cook fish that is one inch thick and about 18 minutes to cook fish that is 1½ inches thick. If you use a meat thermometer on thick pieces of fish, remove the fish from the oven when the thermometer registers a temperature of 150 degrees. (Fish that is not heated above 150 degrees Fahrenheit does not have an oder!)

Garnish fish with chopped parsley and serve with fresh dill, tarragon, chives, lemon juice, or a low-fat sour cream made from yogurt and buttermilk (see Chapter 4).

Steamed Fish

Place the fish on a rack above boiling water. Cover the utensil while the fish cooks. If the fish is one inch thick, steam three to four minutes; if it is two inches thick, steam six to eight minutes. If you use a meat thermometer on thick pieces of fish, do not let the temperature go above 160 degrees.

Fish Patties

1 slightly beaten egg
½ teaspoon salt
1 teaspoon mashed dill seeds
¼ cup wheat germ
1 to 2 cups of steamed or leftover fish

Mix all ingredients, form into patties, and roll in wheat germ. Brown slowly (about eight minutes on each side) in a lightly oiled skillet.

Fish Boats

4 medium (3-ounce) potatoes
16 ounces cooked fish
4 tablespoons hot skim milk
1 teaspoon onion salt

Scrub the potatoes until they are clean, but do not peel. Bake at 425 degrees Fahrenheit for 40 to 50 minutes. When they are done, cut the potatoes in half lengthwise and scoop out their insides. Mash the potato pulp with the fish, hot milk, and onion salt. Then place the mixture in the potato shells. Bake at 400 degrees until brown on top. *Eat the entire potato shell, peel and all.*

Fish in Tomato Sauce

2 tablespoons olive oil
1 onion, finely chopped

1 garlic clove, finely chopped
1 ½ cups chopped ripe tomatoes
salt to taste
1 fresh hot chili pepper, seeded and chopped
¼ teaspoon oregano
1 pound boneless fish

Heat the oil in a saucepan and saute onion and garlic until tender but not brown. Add the tomatoes, parsley, salt, chili pepper, and oregano. Bring to a boil and simmer 20 minutes. Cut the fish into two-inch squares and add to the mixture in the saucepan. Cover and simmer eight minutes or until fish flakes easily.

Salmon Loaf

1 can (1 pound) salmon
1 rib celery, chopped
1 small onion, chopped
1 tablespoon chopped parsley
1 tablespoon wheat germ
1 tablespoon bone meal
1 tablespoon brewer's yeast
1 egg, lightly beaten
1 cup skimmed milk

Preheat oven to 350 degrees. Empty can of salmon into an oiled casserole and add celery, onion, parsley, wheat germ, bone meal, and yeast. Mix the egg and milk and stir into the salmon mixture. Set in a pan of boiling water and bake about one hour.

Shrimp and Rice Casserole

1 scallion with 3 inches green top
1 1-inch cube of cheese
2 tablespoons leftover cooked brown rice
3 ounces cooked shrimp
1 egg
salt and pepper to taste

Chop scallion and grate cheese. Combine scallion, cheese, rice, and shrimp. Beat egg, salt, and pepper together. Fold egg into rice mixture and place in a small, oiled casserole. Set the casserole in a pan of hot water and bake for 25 minutes in an oven preheated to 350 degrees Fahrenheit.

Fish Stew for Two

½ slice slab bacon
1 small onion
½ green pepper
1 stalk celery
1 tomato
2 cups chicken stock or bouillon
1 tablespoon cornmeal
¼ cup water
1 teaspoon brown sugar or honey
1 teaspoon brewer's yeast
1 teaspoon minced dulse
¹⁄₈ teaspoon each of dill, basil, oregano, fennel seed
4 shrimp
3 ounces boneless fish

Cut bacon into ¼-inch pieces and fry. Chop the onion, celery, and green pepper and saute with the bacon. Chop the tomato and add it along with chicken stock to the sauteed vegetables. Add the cornmeal, brown sugar, yeast, dulse, spices, and shrimp. Cover and simmer for 20 minutes. Cut the fish into 1½-inch squares, add to stew, and boil for four minutes.

TASTY EGG DISHES

Boiled eggs are your best bet for a reducing diet, but eggs can be used in a variety of tasty, health-building dishes.

Bacon, Egg, and Potato Casserole

1 slice bacon
½ small tomato
1 scallion with 3 inches green top
1 1-inch cube of cheese
1 teaspoon chopped parsley
2 tablespoons diced boiled potatoes

1 egg
pinch of oregano
salt and pepper to taste

Chop bacon, tomato, and scallion. Fry bacon. Then add tomato and scallion and cook one minute. Combine bacon mixture with parsley, grated cheese, and diced potatoes. Beat egg, oregano, salt, and pepper and add to potato mixture. Place in a small, greased casserole. Set the casserole in a pan of hot water and bake for 25 minutes. Oven should be preheated to 350 degrees.

Sprout and Spinach Scrambled Eggs

1 cup fresh spinach, loosely packed
¼ cup sprouts
1 teaspoon butter
2 eggs
1 1-inch cube of cheese
pinch of basil
salt to taste

Melt the butter in a skillet and add moist spinach. Cover, steam for two minutes, and then shred. Add remaining ingredients to pan and stir until eggs are done.

Eggs Foo Yung

2 tablespoons diced celery
1 tablespoon dehydrated onion flakes
1 tablespoon dehydrated pepper flakes
¼ cup raw sprouts
2 eggs
soy sauce
salt and pepper

Put celery, onion, and pepper into a saucepan and cover with one-half cup of water. Cook until celery is tender (about 15 minutes) and add sprouts. Beat eggs until light, season with salt and pepper, and add vegetable mixture. Drop tablespoons of the batter onto a hot non-stick skillet and brown both sides. Serve with soy sauce.

VARIETY IN VEGETABLES

Steaming is the best way to cook vegetables when you're on a reducing diet. It's sometimes necessary, however, to disguise certain vegetables for the sake of your taste buds.

Skillet Vegetables

1 tablespoon soft margarine
2 cups diagonally sliced carrots
2 cups snap beans, broken into 1-inch pieces
2 cups sliced summer squash
1 cup thinly sliced onion
½ teaspoon salt
black pepper

Melt the margarine in a non-stick skillet. Add the vegetables and the salt. Cover the pan and cook for 10 or 15 minutes or until vegetables are tender. Season with pepper and serve. Yields six servings.

Green Beans with Sprouts

1½ cups green beans
1 strip of bacon
¼ medium-size tomato, diced
pinch of curry and chili powder
½ garlic clove
4 tablespoons water
1 tablespoon alfalfa sprouts

Dice bacon and fry until crisp. Put cut beans into pan and fry in bacon fat for five minutes. Add the tomato, curry, chili powder, garlic, and water and cook over low heat for 15 minutes or until beans are tender. Discard garlic and top with sprouts

Baked Acorn Squash

½ acorn squash
several tablespoons water
2 teaspoons honey
pinch of nutmeg and cloves

Cut squash in half and scoop out seeds. Fill hollow with water, honey, nutmeg, and cloves. Bake for one hour at 350 degrees or until tender.

Cauliflower and Cabbage

1 tablespoon safflower oil
1 teaspoon mustard seeds
1 teaspoon sesame seeds
⅛ teaspoon each of powdered cinnamon, cloves, and cumin
⅛ small head of lettuce
1 cup cauliflower flowerets
¼ teaspoon salt
1 tablespoon yogurt

Heat oil in a skillet. Add mustard seeds, sesame seeds, cinnamon, cloves, and cumin. Stir over medium heat for one minute. Add cauliflower, shredded cabbage, and salt to the skillet and stir-fry for five minutes. Stir in yogurt and simmer for three minutes.

Sprout Salad

Turn back to Chapter 4 and review my method of growing sprouts.

2 large lettuce leaves
½ cup watercress leaves
1 small tomato, chopped
1 tablespoon vinegar
2 teaspoons honey
¼ cup sprouts
salt and pepper to taste

Mix all ingredients together.

Yogurt Dressing

½ cup yogurt
1 egg yolk
¼ teaspoon dry mustard
¼ teaspoon salt

½ teaspoon brown sugar

1 teaspoon lemon juice

Mix all ingredients together and serve as a salad dressing or with cold vegetables or fish.

Tomato and Eggplant Casserole

2 medium-size eggplants
3 tablespoons finely chopped onion
½ teaspoon salt
¼ teaspoon black pepper
1 teaspoon oregano
2 teaspoons soft margarine
4 medium-size tomatoes, sliced
8 ounces Muenster cheese, grated
1 teaspoon paprika

Preheat oven to 350 degrees Fahrenheit. Peel and slice the eggplant. Steam the eggplant in a covered vegetable steamer for 15 minutes. Put the egg plant in a large bowl and mash to a pulp with a fork or a potato masher. Add onion, salt, pepper, and oregano and mix thoroughly. Place the tomato slices in the bottom of a shallow, greased, three-quart baking dish. Spoon the eggplant mixture over the tomatoes and cover with remaining tomato slices. Spread the grated cheese over the tomatoes and sprinkle with paprika. Cover and bake for 45 minutes. Serves five.

Steamed Potatoes

If you do not have time to bake your potatoes, try steaming them.

Leave small potatoes whole and cut large ones in half lengthwise. *Do not peel them.* Your bowels need the fiber supplied by the potato skin. Cook the potatoes by placing them in a covered pot containing one-quarter of a cup of boiling water or by placing them on a rack *above* boiling water. Cook for about 15 minutes or until tender. Salt and pepper to taste.

Corn on the Cob

Corn also provides valuable fiber for your bowels.

Remove outer husks except for a couple of layers next to the corn. Fold the remaining husks back and remove silk. Smear with vegetable oil or soft margarine, sprinkle with salt and pepper, and replace the husks. Place in an oven preheated to 400 degrees and roast for about 12 minutes. If husks are removed, roast for only eight minutes.

To steam corn covered by husks, leave on a covered rack above boiling water for four to six minutes. Steam only three to five minutes if husks are removed.

Cooked Green Beans

Cut beans into two-inch pieces and put into a shallow pan with one-half cup of salted water. Bring to a boil and then cover pan and simmer for 10 to 12 minutes. Beans should be done but still green and crisp.

BREADS AND CEREALS

In Chapter 4, I gave you a recipe for bran-rich whole-wheat bread. In order to put a little additional bran in your diet, use these recipes occasionally. Remember that you need all the bran and fiber you can get (from natural foods) for healthy bowels as well as to hinder absorption of calories.

Bran Muffins

1 cup coarse unprocessed bran flakes
1 cup whole-wheat pastry flour
1 teaspoon salt
1 teaspoon cinnamon
2 tablespoons vegetable oil
1 cup skimmed milk
4 eggs (separated)
3 tablespoons honey
½ cup raisins

Mix bran flakes, flour, salt, and cinnamon. In another bowl, combine oil, milk, raisins, beaten egg yolks, and honey; add to flour mixture. Beat the egg whites stiff and fold into the batter. Bake in oiled muffin tins at 375 degrees for 30 minutes.

Corn Pone

3 cups white cornmeal
⅓ cup sesame seeds
a few caraway seeds
½ teaspoon salt
¼ cup corn oil
several cups of boiling water

Mix the meal, sesame seeds, and the salt. Pour in the corn oil and water. Mix and form into patties. Bake in a 350-degree oven for about 50 minutes.

Corn Bread

If you do not like coarse corn pone, try this recipe.

3 cups cornmeal
2 teaspoons baking powder
1 teaspoon baking soda
1½ teaspoons salt
2 cups buttermilk
3 eggs, slightly beaten

Mix the cornmeal, baking powder, baking soda, and salt. Add the buttermilk and eggs. Bake in a 425-degree oven for 25 to 30 minutes. (Use a shallow pan if you want crisp corn bread.)

Vigor Cereal

There are many good natural cereals on the market, but many of them tend to be too sweet. You can make your own to suit your taste.

¼ cup wheat germ
½ cup rolled oats
2 tablespoons rice polish
¼ cup flaked wheat
¼ cup flaked rye
6 dates
¼ cup raisins
¼ cup sunflower seeds
¼ cup almonds
1 tablespoon soy powder
¼ cup coconut meal

Place the wheat germ, rolled oats, rice polish, flaked wheat, and flaked rye in a glass baking dish and bake for 10 minutes in an oven preheated to 250 degrees. Heap this mixture and the dates on a chopping board and chop to bits. Stir in the remaining ingredients and store in a mason jar.

Wheat Germ Muffins

1 cup sifted whole-wheat pastry flour
1 teaspoon salt
3 teaspoons baking powder
¼ cup powdered milk
1 cup wheat germ
1 cup milk
2 eggs
¼ cup honey
2 tablespoons vegetable oil
½ cup raisins

Put flour, salt, baking powder, and powdered milk into bowl and mix. Stir in the remaining ingredients. Fill greased muffin tins two-thirds full and bake at 400 degrees Fahrenheit for 15 to 20 minutes or until brown.

MISCELLANEOUS RECIPES

Cottage Cheese Pancakes

You shouldn't eat pancakes very often. But when you do, cottage cheese pancakes will provide protein and other essential nutrients.

½ cup cottage cheese
1 teaspoon safflower oil
2 tablespoons whole-wheat flour
1 tablespoon raw sugar
1 egg
1 teaspoon wheat germ
½ teaspoon brewer's yeast
4 pecan halves, chopped
½ teaspoon sesame seeds
⅛ teaspoon each of cinnamon and salt

3 teaspoons yogurt
3 teaspoons honey

Beat all ingredients together except for the yogurt and the honey. Form six pancakes on an oiled baking sheet. Sprinkle with cinnamon and bake 25 minutes in an oven preheated to 350 degrees. Spread each pancake with one-half teaspoon of yogurt and one-half teaspoon of honey.

Vegetable Soup

You can make your own vegetable soup with any combination of your favorite vegetables. Here's a sample recipe.

6 cups boiling water or tomato juice
3 tablespoons rolled oats
1 tablespoon rice polishings
2 cups chopped tomatoes
1 bay leaf
salt to taste
1½ cups shredded cabbage
1½ cups chopped celery
½ cup sliced green beans
½ cup fresh peas
½ teaspoon marjoram
2 tablespoons chopped parsley
½ cup cooked brown rice
1 cup shredded escarole

Combine the boiling water or tomato juice with the oats and the rice polishings and cook until thick. Then add the remaining ingredients, except the escarole, and cook in a covered pot for about 15 minutes, until the vegetables are tender. Add the escarole and cook three minutes longer. If you want to make a complete meal of vegetable soup, add tuna or shrimp.

Soy Milk

To make soy milk, blend one quart of water with one cup of soy flour and one-quarter cup of calcium lactate. If you desire, you can flavor the milk with one teaspoon of vanilla and two teaspoons of honey. Boil over low heat for 10 minutes. Strain if necessary.

Your local health food store can supply you with the ingredients and the instructions you need to make soy milk and other soy dishes.

SUMMARY

1. Use simple cooking methods to prepare the foods of a reducing diet, with an occasional "combination recipe" for variety.

2. Health-food recipes provide a good opportunity to include bone meal, brewer's yeast, wheat germ, and other nutritious supplements in cooking.

3. Even if you are no longer overweight, you should continue to use natural-food recipes to build good health.

4. Any recipe can be altered to suit your taste—or you may even make up your own recipes.

5. With a little imagination, you can mix up a "one meal" dish that can serve as a complete, balanced meal.

6. Meats, fish, and poultry should always be cooked slowly at a low temperature to preserve juiciness and tenderness.

7. Recipes calling for soybeans can be used instead of meat recipes.

8. Vegetables that you do not enjoy eating can be made more appetizing by combining them with other foods or by flavoring them with herbs and broths.

9. You can add important fiber to your diet by eating whole-grain breads and cereals prepared at home.

10. Expand your knowledge of selecting and preparing natural foods by studying natural-foods cookbooks.

11

How to Enjoy
Delicious Fat-Fighting Treats

If you're really serious about reducing your bodyweight, you won't eat nonessential treats very often. You'll satisfy your appetite with fresh, natural foods that supply essential fat-fighting nutrients. Fresh and dried fruits, nuts, cheese, and whole-grain crackers, for example, are good health-building treats. Few of us can completely eliminate nonessential snacks, however, especially sweets. If you'll limit your sweets to nutritious *natural* sweets, there's no reason why you cannot occasionally treat your sweet tooth, especially if you are no longer overweight.

IT'S A MATTER OF TASTE

If you are not accustomed to eating sweets, you may not care for them. If not, you should continue to avoid all sweets except fresh and dried fruits. If you do crave sweets, you should make a special effort to avoid *refined* sweets (made with white sugar and other artificial ingredients) and eat only *natural* sweets. Once you have developed a taste for natural sweets, you'll lose your taste for refined sweets, and your appetite mechanism will function more efficiently. Best of all, you'll be healthier and leaner.

MAKE YOUR OWN SWEETS

First try to satisfy your craving for sweets with fresh and dried fruits. If you feel that you *must* have something sweeter, you can make your own sweets with all-natural ingredients. This will at least assure that you get the nutrients you need to *combat* a craving for sweets. Using raisins or honey as a sweetener, for example, keeps a snack within a health-building category. And if a natural sweet keeps you away from processed snacks, it can also be classified as a fat-fighting snack.

You should, of course, limit your use of sweets, even if they are natural and you are not overweight. As a rule, it usually takes only a small amount of any natural sweet to satisfy your craving. A half teaspoon of honey, for example, will satisfy anyone's sweet tooth. Artificial sweets, on the other hand, will artificially *stimulate* your appetite for sweets as well as deprive you of nutrients.

It's important to remember that even natural sweets are high in calories. Honey is just as rich in calories as white sugar. This means that you can build an excessive amount of body fat with sweets of any type if you eat too much. The difference is that natural sweets contain nutrients, and they satisfy your appetite more readily.

Eat Sweets Only After a Regular Meal

When you do eat sweets, eat them only after a regular meal, when your appetite has been satisfied with fresh, natural foods. It's true that snacking on sweets will reduce your appetite so that you'll eat less at mealtime. But on a health-building, fat-disintegrator diet, you *need* the nutrients supplied by a balanced diet if you are to eliminate the craving that forces you to eat an excessive amount of fat-building sweets. So eat your sweets *last,* and then eat only a small amount.

Between-meal snacks should consist of fruit, cheese, broiled chicken, raw vegetables, and other natural foods that supply essential nutrients. Then, when you eat smaller meals, you won't be depriving yourself of adequate nutrients.

Nonsweet "Desserts"

I have found that a piece of fruit with a few raisins, or a piece of cheese, or a small piece of crisp corn pone, is a satisfying way to end a meal. And it leaves a clean, fresh taste in my mouth. If you don't crave sweets, don't eat them. There may be a better way for you to finish a meal. But if you do crave sweets, eat *natural* sweets so that you won't attempt to satisfy your craving by eating an excessive amount of other types of foods.

RECIPES FOR HEALTH-BUILDING SWEETS AND SNACKS

There are endless combinations and varieties of natural foods that can serve as health-building snacks or desserts. Here are a few. In your search for new recipes, first make sure that what you eat will improve your health. Use the low-calorie recipes most often. Go easy on the high-calorie recipes.

Carob Carrot Bran Cake

In Chapter 10, I gave you a recipe for bran muffins to put a little fiber in your diet. Here's a recipe for a delicious, health-building *dessert* that will also supply valuable fiber.

½ cup raisins
¾ cup whole-wheat flour
¼ cup soy flour
½ cup bran flakes
3 tablespoons carob flour
1½ teaspoons cinnamon
2 teaspoons grated orange or lemon rind
¼ teaspoon salt
1 cup grated carrots
2 eggs, separated

Put the raisins in a cup and add hot water until the cup is full. Pour the contents of the cup into a bowl and add the remaining ingredients except for the egg whites. Beat the egg whites until they are stiff and fold into the mixture in the bowl.

Place in an oiled bread pan and bake at 350 degrees F. for about 55 minutes. Delicious with yogurt.

Carob "Candy"

If you like the taste of chocolate, you'll like carob. You can prepare this recipe without doing any cooking.

½ cup carob powder
½ cup honey
½ cup unhydrogenated peanut butter
½ cup sunflower seeds
½ cup sesame seeds
½ cup wheat germ
¼ cup soy powder

Mix all ingredients and form into balls. Roll in chopped, unsweetened coconut.

Note: Carob comes from a pod that grows on a tree. It has a naturally sweet chocolate flavor. If your local grocery store doesn't have any carob powder, you can find some in a health food store.

Sesame Seed Cookies

6 tablespoons sesame seed butter
½ cup honey
½ cup chopped walnuts or peanuts
1½ cups oatmeal
½ teaspoon cinnamon

Sesame seed butter, also called tahini, is made by putting sesame seeds in a blender and reducing them to a butter.

Mix honey and sesame seed butter together and then mix in remaining ingredients. (Also delicious with chopped apples, raisins, or dates.) Drop mixture onto oiled cookie sheet with a spoon and bake at 350 degrees F. for about 10 minutes or until edges are brown.

Note: Your local health food store can supply you with ready-made sesame seed butter or tahini.

Tahini Treats

Here's another dessert recipe that does not require cooking.

½ cup finely ground coconut, unsweetened
½ cup sunflower seed meal
½ cup wheat germ
¼ cup sesame seed butter
¼ cup honey

Mix all ingredients together and divide into two portions.
Roll each portion into a one-inch cylinder (in wax paper) and
keep in the refrigerator. Cut servings as needed.

Raw Peanut Butter Candy

½ cup unhydrogenated peanut butter
½ cup honey
1 cup powdered milk

Mix the peanut butter and honey and stir in the powdered
milk. Add nuts or shredded coconut if desired. Place on buttered
wax paper and cut into squares or form into a roll, chill, and cut
into slices.

Note: Natural or unhydrogenated peanut butter can be
found in any health food store.

Stuffed Dates and Prunes

Stuff pitted dates or prunes with raw nuts. A combination
of dried fruits and nuts makes a delicious substitute for candy. A
date stuffed with a pecan half is one of my favorite desserts.

Wheat Germ Oatmeal Cookies

¾ cup vegetable oil
1¼ cups honey
2 eggs
2 teaspoons vanilla
1 cup raisins or ½cup each of chopped nuts and raisins
1½ cups wheat germ
2 cups rolled oats
¾ cup whole-wheat flour
1 teaspoon salt
½ cup powdered milk

Sift in the flour, salt, and milk *after* mixing all the other ingredients. Stir until mixed well. Form cookies on a lightly oiled baking sheet and bake at 350 degrees F. for 10 to 12 minutes.

Peanut Butter and Sunflower Seed Celery

When you need a health-building snack that's not sweet, try this tasty recipe. Peanut butter makes a good between-meal snack for persons who suffer from hypoglycemia or low blood sugar.

2 8-inch celery stalks without leaves
2 tablespoons unhydrogenated peanut butter
1 teaspoon wheat germ
1 tablespoon sunflower seeds
⅛ teaspoon salt

Mix the peanut butter, wheat germ, and salt and stuff into celery Cut each stuffed celery in half and sprinkle with sunflower seeds.

Chicken and Cheese Balls

This tasty and nutritious snack will help curb your appetite at mealtime.

¼ cup chopped, cooked chicken breast
1 1-inch cube of cheese, grated
2 teaspoons grated onion
⅛ teaspoon curry powder
⅛ teaspoon salt
1 tablespoon wheat germ
10 watercress leaves

Mash the chicken and cheese together. Add the onion, curry powder, and salt. Mix, form into 10 balls, and roll in wheat germ. Spear a watercress leaf to each ball with a toothpick.

Fruit Spread Sandwiches

Serve this spread on one-half slices of homemade whole-grain bread.

1 small pear
1 apple
2 tablespoons raisins

1½ tablespoons honey
1 teaspoon wheat germ

Remove the seeds, core, and stem of the pear and the apple. Grate the fruit, chop the raisins, and mix all ingredients together.

Cold Curry Sauce

Dip raw vegetable strips into this spicy sauce for a tasty appetizer.

½ cup yogurt
2 teaspoons honey
½ teaspoon lemon juice
¼ teaspoon curry powder
1 tablespoon chopped pumpkin seeds

Mix all ingredients together and chill.

Strawberry Yogurt

This cold, refreshing yogurt dish can be substituted for ice cream.

1 cup yogurt
1 cup fresh, ripe strawberries
2 tablespoons honey

Freeze the yogurt in a refrigerator tray. Puree the strawberries and honey in a blender. Beat the frozen yogurt into the puree and freeze in a refrigerator tray.

Frozen Strawberry Cream

Serve this frozen delight over fresh fruit or as a dessert.

1 cup whole, ripe strawberries
2 tablespoons honey
¾ cup cottage cheese

Mix all ingredients in a blender. Divide into two small dishes and freeze. Stir with a fork and freeze again. Remove from the freezer just before serving.

Frozen Prune Whip

Prunes aren't just for "old folks." They're delicious alone or in desserts.

8 dried, pitted prunes
½ cup water
½ apple, cored
3 tablespoons cottage cheese
2 tablespoons honey
2 tablespoons yogurt
⅛ teaspoon cinnamon

Soak the prunes in the water for one hour. Then simmer the prunes in the soaking water until there are about two tablespoons of syrup in the bottom of the pot. Chop the apple. Put the apple, the prunes, the syrup, the cottage cheese, and the honey into a blender and mix well. Stir the yogurt and cinnamon into the prune mixture and freeze until mushy. Beat the frozen mixture with a fork until it is fluffy. Spoon into individual containers and refreeze. Remove from the freezer just before serving.

Vegetable Drink

Any fruit or vegetable juice can serve as a refreshing party beverage. This combination of vegetable juices can double as a low-calorie beverage and a health cocktail.

½ cup tomato juice
¼ cup celery juice
¼ cup carrot juice
¼ bunch watercress, chopped
1 teaspoon chopped parsley
1 teaspoon lemon juice
2 teaspoons brewer's yeast

Mix all ingredients in an electric blender. Chill before serving. Yields two servings.

Orange-Prune Drink

If you dread your morning or evening prune juice, you'll appreciate this drink.

⅓ cup orange juice
⅓ cup unsweetened prune juice
2 teaspoons honey

1 teaspoon wheat germ
2 ice cubes

Mix all ingredients in a blender and serve immediately.

Cranberry-Orange Drink

The acid residue supplied by this cold, refreshing drink will help keep your kidneys healthy.

⅔ cup orange juice
¼ cup fresh cranberries
1 tablespoon honey
2 ice cubes
1 tablespoon yogurt

Mix all ingredients in a blender until smooth and foamy. Serve immediately.

Yogurt Dip

Instead of serving questionable processed cheese dips to family and friends, improve their health with this yogurt dip.

6 walnut halves
1 garlic clove
1 tablespoon olive oil
1 cup yogurt
¼ cup diced cucumber
½ teaspoon lemon juice
whole-grain crackers

Mash walnuts, garlic, and oil to a paste (or mix in a blender). Stir the mixture into the yogurt along with the cucumber and the lemon juice. Chill and serve with whole-grain crackers. Serves four.

Party Cheese Dip

There's no substitute for the taste of Cheddar cheese, especially in combination with tomatoes.

½ pound shredded Cheddar cheese
1½ cups chopped ripe tomatoes
1 tablespoon chopped hot green chili pepper
carrot sticks

scallions
cauliflowerets
zucchini sticks
cucumber sticks

Place cheese and tomatoes in a saucepan and neat gently until cheese is melted. Add chili pepper and serve with raw vegetable dippers Serves six.

SUMMARY

1. Sweet desserts should be kept to a minimum on a fat-disintegrator or fat-fighting diet.

2. Refined sweets should be avoided completely!

3. Whenever possible, your sweet tooth should be satisfied with fresh and dried fruits.

4. It's best to make your own sweets with all-natural ingredients.

5. Although natural sweets contain health-building nutrients, they should be eaten sparingly if you are overweight.

6. Eat sweets and desserts only *after* a regular noon or evening meal.

7. Nutritious, low-calorie snacks may be eaten between meals in order to curb your appetite at mealtime.

8. Do your family and your friends a favor and serve them natural low-calorie snacks and homemade sweets made with all-natural ingredients.

9. Delicious, natural, health-building beverages can be served as a treat as well as during a regular meal.

10. The recipes in this chapter will give you some idea of the type of recipes you should use to prepare treats and desserts.

12

Questions and Answers about Sensible Eating and Safe Reducing

This chapter, in the form of questions and answers, will answer many questions left unanswered in previous chapters. It will also help summarize what you have learned from reading this book. When you want to review the basic rules of my fat-disintegrator and fat-fighting diets, read the summaries at the end of each chapter. Then read these questions and answers to test your knowledge of sensible eating and safe reducing.

Why do most doctors recommend that you lose only two or three pounds a week?

Answer: Rapid weight loss can result in undesirable side effects. Also, any diet that results in a loss of several pounds a week is likely to be deficient in the nutrients needed to prevent disease in an overweight body. It would be best to consume enough food to prevent loss of more than a few pounds a week. Then, as your body becomes lighter, you can progressively reduce your calorie intake to assure continued weight loss. If you lose only two pounds a week, you can lose 96 pounds in a year! What more could you ask for?

How do you determine how much to eat to keep from losing weight?

Answer: Generally speaking, you need about 15 calories a day to maintain each pound of the *existing* bodyweight. If you eat strictly natural foods, it's likely that your bodyweight will *normalize* when it reaches a level that's best for you. Looking in the mirror or stepping on the scales can guide you in reducing or increasing the amount of food you eat.

I have a friend who is losing 10 pounds a week on some kind of a diet, and he looks healthy to me. Couldn't I try his diet for a couple of weeks?

Answer: Quick weight loss usually means that the body is losing water, which returns when the diet is discontinued. Since you cannot stay on an unbalanced diet for very long, weight loss on such a diet is always temporary. The only kind of diet that you can follow for a lifetime is one that results in a slow and gradual loss of weight. A natural-foods diet, such as my fat-disintegrator diet, is a lifetime diet that results in an automatic adjustment in weight.

Why are baked potatoes allowed on a fat-disintegrator diet? I have always heard that potatoes are fattening.

Answer: Potatoes are not as fattening as most people think. One medium baked potato contains only 93 calories, less than a serving of lean beef. Potatoes contain all the nutrients your body needs to metabolize the carbohydrate they contain. Since a potato is a *natural carbohydrate*, your appetite mechanism will not allow you to eat more than your body can use—provided you eat baked or boiled potatoes rather than fried or "dressed up" potatoes.

I went to a doctor who told me that I have low blood sugar and that I am sensitive to carbohydrates. Does this mean that I should not eat potatoes?

Answer: *Refined* carbohydrates are usually responsible for blood sugar problems that lead to overweight. If you eat nothing but natural foods, including potatoes, it's not likely that you'll have any trouble with your blood sugar. If you find from experience, however, that weight loss is too slow on a balanced diet of natural foods, it may be necessary to restrict the use of potatoes and other carbohydrate-rich foods until your weight is down.

My husband and I eat the same things, but I get fat while he stays slim. Do you think it has something to do with my hormones?

Answer: Regular physical activity usually keeps big eaters slim. In addition to burning calories, physical activity conditions the muscles to dispose of excess calories 24 hours a day. This means that once muscles have been trained, their constant metabolic activity burns calories even while you are resting!

Once you are physically fit, it takes only about 10 or 15 minutes of exercise twice a week to stay in shape. If you want to eat more and look better, get a little regular exercise in some form of recreational activity.

I've been exercising regularly and following your fat-disintegrator diet for three weeks. I look better, and I've lost inches, but my scales do not show any weight loss. Why is this?

Answer: While exercise burns off excess body fat, it also develops muscles. If your muscles are small and weak, exercise will make them larger and stronger. As the fat melts away, it may be replaced by muscle to some extent. Persons who are only moderately overweight may not experience much weight loss during the first six weeks of a combined exercise and reducing program. The result, however, is a tremendous improvement in physical appearance. Continued use of a diet-exercise program will result in loss of excess body fat and a reduction in bodyweight.

Muscles will not get any larger after several weeks of regular physical activity. A small amount of exercise a couple of times a week, however, will greatly speed weight loss by stimulating metabolic activity in the muscles.

Many low-calorie recipes call for sauteing with vegetable oil. Doesn't the oil add extra calories?

Answer: Any kind of oil is high in calories. A tablespoonful of vegetable oil, for example, contains about 124 calories, compared with 93 in a medium-size baked potato. You need some oil in your diet, however, since it supplies essential fatty acids and helps satisfy your appetite. If you use a couple of tablespoons of vegetable oil daily on salads, or if you use a small amount of soft margarine on toast, you'll get all the oil you need. You can eliminate the use of oil in sauteing and frying by using teflon pans with a little water, bouillon, or chicken stock. When you are sauteing vegetables, for example, just keep adding a little water while stirring the vegetables.

Are natural sweets as fattening as refined sweets?

Answer: Natural sweets that are high in calories can contribute to a build-up of body fat, but not as readily as refined sweets. Natural sweets, such as fresh and dried fruits, contain a more complex form of carbohydrate (sugar) and are digested and absorbed more slowly than refined sweets. This means that the blood sugar will not be elevated suddenly to *force* the storage of blood sugar as fat. So while you should *never* eat refined or commercial sweets, you may eat natural sweets if you eat them sparingly in a balanced diet.

Why do most reducing diets recommend that you eat fish?

Answer: Fish is rich in protein and low in fat, and the fat it does contain is largely unsaturated. Even if you aren't overweight, the essential fatty acids in fish help prevent a build-up of hard fat in your arteries.

All fats contain calories, but the fattest or oiliest fish contains fewer calories than most meats. If you eat a variety of fish, you don't have to worry about how much fat the fish contains. Mackerel and salmon are fairly high in calories, so they should be your last choice.

You should never eat sardines or tuna canned in oil. If you cannot find these fish packed in water or tomato sauce, wash away the oil before eating them.

If you want to know more about how to prepare fish, order *Let's Cook Fish* (60¢), #8, from the Superintendent of Documents, U.S. Government Printing Office, Washington, D.C. 20402.

How do you know how much protein, carbohydrate, and fat you must have for good health?

Answer: Nutritionists tell us that about 25 percent of the food we eat should be protein. Every diet should contain *at least* 60 grams of carbohydrate (about 43 percent in a balanced diet), with about 30 percent of the calorie requirement being supplied by fat. And in order to protect your heart and your arteries, there should be about two parts vegetable fat to one part animal fat.

If you follow a balanced diet, such as my fat-disintegrator diet, you don't have to worry about measuring portions of protein, carbohydrate, and fat. You'll automatically get the correct amounts of the essential food elements if you'll eat the recommended basic foods.

A reducing diet that's deliberately unbalanced so that it's deficient in carbohydrate or too rich in protein or fat can have harmful effects that may permanently damage your health. So don't be too anxious to try a zero-carbohydrate diet, a high-protein diet, or a high-fat diet, all of which result in weight loss because of a deficiency in nutrients.

What about using non-stick sprays in cooking?

Answer: Sprays containing vegetable oil and lecithin are often used to coat the inside of pots and pans so that foods won't stick to the utensils during cooking. Such sprays are perfectly safe to use and will help cut down on the use of oil in baking and frying. Lecithin and vegetable oil are natural substances, and as a spray they'll transmit fewer calories than oil or grease that can be soaked up by the food being cooked. Vegetable oil sprays used with non-stick utensils will eliminate the need for cooking oil in frying.

Why is prime meat often not recommended in a reducing diet?

Answer: In addition to being expensive, prime meats have more fat than cheaper meats. Marbling in steak, for example, is fat that makes the steak juicy and tasty. Cheaper cuts of meat usually have less marbling and therefore less fat. Since you should cut away all the fat from the meat you eat, don't waste your money on prime cuts. You can't cut away the marbling in fat meats, and you don't need the calories and the cholesterol found in such meats. Buy the leaner, cheaper meats, and then ask your butcher to cut away all the visible fat.

Does toasted bread have fewer calories than fresh bread?

Answer: Toasting bread does *not* decrease its calorie content. A slice of whole-wheat bread contains about 60 calories. If you make your own bread, you can *reduce absorption* of calories by adding bran to increase the fiber content of the bread.

Gluten bread (made from high-protein flour) contains only about 35 calories a slice. Remember, however, that you need the Vitamin E and the fiber supplied by whole-grain breads and cereals. If you limit your bread to one slice at each meal and eat only natural, whole-grain bread, you don't have to worry about the calories in bread.

Can cold cuts be a part of a reducing diet?

Answer: Some cold cuts may be low in calories; but since they usually contain artificial additives, I do not recommend them. Preservatives and other additives may have harmful effects in the body. Some may even cause cancer. Processed cheese packaged foods, and other "unnatural foods" may also contain additives. If you want to be healthy as well as slim, stick to fresh, natural foods.

Which is more fattening, margarine or butter?

Answer: Margarine and butter are equally fattening, since both contain the same number of calories. A tablespoonful of each contains about 100 calories.

If you have to choose between pure butter and hard margarine, you should always choose the butter. When margarine has been totally hardened by a process called hydrogenation, it is a *hard fat* that can be more damaging to your arteries than butter, since it does not contain all the nutrients found in butter. *Soft* margarine, which has been only partially hydrogenated, is rich in the soft vegetable oil you need to prevent a build-up of hard fat in your arteries. So while you may use small amounts of butter and soft margarine, you should avoid hard margarine.

If eggs are not fattening, how can they damage your arteries?

Answer: Eggs are a good source of protein, Vitamin A, and other nutrients. The yolk of an egg, however, is rich in cholesterol, a waxy substance that tends to clog arteries. Since cholesterol is not a fat, it does not contribute to a build-up of body fat. If you do not have a high blood cholesterol, there's no reason why you cannot eat eggs freely in a balanced reducing diet.

One medium egg supplies about 81 calories, about 60 of which are in the yolk. You need the nutrients supplied by the yolk of an egg. But if you eat an excessive number of eggs, you may have to eliminate some of the yolk.

Some reducing diets are called "low-carbohydrate diets," and some are called "low-fat diets." Which is most fattening, carbohydrate or fat?

Answer: Low-carbohydrate diets restrict the use of vegetables, fruits, grains, breads, and cereals and allow unlimited use of meats and fats. Low-fat diets restrict the use of fats, oils, meats, and other foods rich in fat. Both diets result in a reduction in bodyweight, since the overall effect is a reduction in the number of calories consumed. Too little carbohydrate or fat in the diet, however, can have harmful effects.

Generally speaking, fat is richest in calories. Fat supplies nine calories per gram, while protein and carbohydrate each supply four calories per gram. Since fat contributes the most calories and may have a damaging effect on blood vessels, it's best to go easy on fat and depend more upon natural carbohydrates for calories (energy).

An excessive amount of protein may also be harmful. A diet that's too low in carbohydrate is likely to be too high in fat and protein.

Note: *Refined* carbohydrates are extremely fattening and are responsible for most of the obesity in the United States. Eliminating refined carbohydrates and keeping natural carbohydrates in proper proportion to protein and fat is the secret of a successful, *healthful* reduction in bodyweight.

Measuring foods in terms of cups and ounces is confusing to me. Could you give me a table of measurements commonly used in reducing diets?

Answer: For measuring the *volume* of food, use this table:

1 cup equals 8 ounces or ½ pint or 16 tablespoons
2 tablespoons equals 1 fluid ounce
1 pint equals 2 cups
1 quart equals 4 cups

You can purchase a measuring cup that has the ounces marked on the side of the cup for easy measuring.

To measure the *weight* of food, use this table:

1 ounce equals 28.35 grams
100 grams equals 3½ ounces
16 ounces equals 1 pound

Can you eat too much meat?

Answer: Although some reducing diets stress extensive use of lean meats, a diet of too much meat, like any unbalanced diet, can be harmful. An excessive amount of protein overloads the kidneys, contributes to the development of gout, and creates a calcium deficiency. Protein also contributes calories that can be stored as fat. Unless you are an athlete or a bodybuilder doing heavy resistance exercise, it's not necessary that your diet be made up of more than 25 percent protein.

Remember that even lean meats contain a considerable amount of invisible fat and cholesterol. This is why persons who are overweight or who have atherosclerosis are advised to eat chicken or fish rather than meat.

When my weight is back to normal, can I start eating sugar again?

Answer: If possible, you should swear off white sugar forever. The average American consumes about 115 pounds of sugar a year. This figures out to about 500 calories a day, which is equivalent to adding one pound of body fat a week. This means that most of us could lose 48 pounds in a year simply by eliminating sugar.

If you eat strictly natural foods, you won't be consuming the hidden sugar in processed or packaged foods. With no sugar or artificial foods in your diet, you can eat more of the natural foods that build good health and fight fat.

Does the amount of water you drink have anything to do with bodyweight?

Answer: If your body is healthy, it will take the water it needs and eliminate the rest. Drinking large amounts of water will not add fat to your body. When you are reducing your bodyweight, however, you should go easy on the use of table salt so that your tissues won't retain the water released by the combustion of fat. During the first few weeks of any reducing diet, the body may be reluctant to release water leftover when fat is burned for energy. This is why weight loss may be slow at first.

Will steam baths, saunas, vibrators, and massage help reduce body fat?

Answer: No! Fat must be burned for energy if bodyweight is to be reduced. The only way this can be accomplished is by dieting or by exercising. Combining diet and exercise is the best way to reduce body fat if you want to eat generously.

Weight lost in a steam bath is only water, which is quickly replaced.

CONCLUSION

Even after you have successfully reduced your bodyweight, you should continue to follow the guidelines of this book. The use of natural foods in your daily diet will add many healthy years to your life.

Anyone can follow the basic recommendations of this book with equally good results. So don't hesitate to recommend my fat-disintegrator diet to your family and your friends.

As the years go by, you'll want to refer to this book frequently to refresh your knowledge of selecting and preparing natural foods. With continued attention to what you eat each day, you'll never again be fat.

Index